MMS Protocols

Book Two

MMS Protocols

MMS Protocols

Book Two

Rev. Dr. May

3

MMS Protocols

Published and Distributed in The United States by: Star Rising Publishers.

Library of Congress Cataloging-in-Publication Data

May, Rev. Dr.
MMS Protocols Book Two / Rev. Dr. May

ISBN-13: 978-1893774605
Tradepaper: ISBN: 978-1893774605

1st edition, June 2011

STAR RISING PUBLISHERS
Printed in The United States of America

Book Two

MMS Protocols

Contents

MMS Protocols

Book Two

MMS Protocols

MMS Explained

The Miracle Mineral Supplement (MMS) is a very effective solution for many ailments. MMS often works in a few hours. It destroys malaria in just 4 hours. The patient often resumes work the next day.

The immune system uses MMS to attack germs, bacteria, viruses, molds, and other microorganisms that are harmful to the body. It will not affect friendly bacteria, including intestinal flora. MMS also leaves healthy cells untouched.

MMS is the greatest solution against diseases and ills now known, and it is not a drug.

MMS is the purest of all things that you might take. Drugs and even nutrients have dozens of different combinations of chemicals and different elements. That's generally the reason for the side effects associated with them. Look at any drug formula. Often the formula listing is longer than a foot. MMS is only two simple items once dissolved in water. MMS consists of the type of harmless chlorine that is in table salt, and oxygen. There is some sodium, before it is dissolved in the water, but that becomes harmless because it is only a trace amount.

This combination results in the most powerful killer of pathogens known. It has been used in stock yards to kill pathogens on meat, and on slaughtered chickens; it has been used to sterilize hospital floors and benches, and to kill pathogens in water works without killing friendly bacteria for over 70 years.

Now this same formula is used in the body, and the same situation results. No damage is done to the body, but the pathogens are destroyed. In its powerful form MMS is chlorine dioxide that reverts back to harmless chloride and neutralized oxygen. It leaves nothing behind to build up in the body.

Technically Speaking

MMS is not chlorine dioxide; MMS is sodium chlorite $(NaClO2)$ 28%, Actually 22.4%. Combining with acid briefly produces chlorous acid $(HClO2)$, which in sequential steps oxidizes ambient chlorite $(ClO2-)$ to create chlorine dioxide $(ClO2)$.

Common Uses

Activated MMS is a biocide which means it selects only pathogens that may be harmful to humans and larger animals. Chlorine dioxide's powerful sanitizing qualities, combined with its lack of toxicity and mutagenicity, make MMS products the ideal solutions for an extensive list of animal health-related applications, including treatment of skin infections, wounds, scratches and lacerations, ear-cleaning agent and treatment for otitis externa in dogs and cats caused by bacteria, yeast agent and treatment for otitis externa in dogs and cats caused by bacteria, yeast and viral infections, treatment of hoof abscess, white line disease, thrush, hoof canker and other dermatophytosis; antiseptic shampoo cleans and deodorizes hair coat and skin, eliminates dandruff and skunk odors, treatment of dermatitis and dermatological "hot spots" in all animals, treatment of fungal and yeast infections, treatment of abscesses, surgical site prep, after normal surgical prep, cold sterilization of surgical equipment, and dental paste helps eliminate bacteria responsible for peritonitis and gingivitis and whitens stained teeth. It is even used to cold sterilize surgical instruments.

Proper Way to Store MMS

MMS should be stored in a dark cabinet that is moderate in temperature, no extremes. An ideal location that many people choose is a cabinet in the kitchen that is not opened frequently.

Citric acid solution that is already mixed may be kept in the refrigerator to prolong the life of the product, though not necessary. MMS should NOT be kept in the refrigerator because of the interior light that comes on when the door is opened. MMS is sensitive to light and the MMS may lose it's potency.

Heat extremes will cause MMS to expand and may cause leakage from the top of the bottle. If it is in plastic bottle the bottle may burst. Keep MMS out of direct sunlight as this too

MMS Protocols

will cause the MMS to expand and burst.

MMS Protocols

In this section there are several different protocols for taking MMS. All of them are correct and all of them will give you the same end result, it is just a matter of how fast or how slow you want to proceed. If you have a sensitive system proceed slower. If you are treating something terminal then go faster. Always adjust your intake according to the amount you can tolerate.

Updated Main Protocol

The main protocol is basically taking 3 drops of activated MMS each hour, for 8 hours a day, for 3 weeks. However many people cannot start taking that many drops and should start with only 2 or even 1 drop and hour. This is determined by how sick they are to begin with. If one is feeling very sick then start with 1 drop an hour or even 1/2 drop and hour, but then begin taking more if you feel that you can. The rule is, if you feel that the drops are making you feel worse, take less and if they are not making you feel worse then take a little bit more the next hour, but never more than 3 drops an hour.

The way you accomplish activation can be done in 4 different

17

ways, any one of these methods of activation is acceptable: First, add your number of MMS drops to a clean dry glass, then activate as follows:

(1) (preferred method) add 1 drop of 50% citric acid for each drop of MMS that is in your glass, swirl or shake to mix, wait 20 seconds, add 1/2 to 1 glass of water or juice and drink.
(2) add 5 drops of 10% citric acid for each drop of MMS in the glass, and then swirl to mix, wait 3 minutes, add 1/2 to 1 glass of water or juice and then drink.

(3) add 5 drops of vinegar for each drop of MMS in the glass, shake or swirl to mix, wait 3 minutes, add 1/2 to 1 glass of water or juice and then drink.

(4) add 5 drops of full strength lemon juice for each drop of MMS in the glass, shake or swirl to mix, add 1/2 to 1 glass of water or juice and then drink.

Do not use orange juice. Do not use juices with added vitamin C or ascorbic acid added. Do not use concentrated juices that must have water added to them. Fresh juices are best.

But if you do not want to make up a single dose each hour, you can make 8 doses in the morning, and keep the solution in a closed container all day. Just follow the above instructions multiplying all the figures by 8 and then put that liquid in a closed container. Take 1/8th of it each hour. Do not worry the MMS will last hours longer than is needed.

Important instructions: do not make yourself sicker than you already are. Do not cause yourself a lot of nausea, pain, or diarrhea. When you notice any of these symptoms coming on take less MMS. Try not to stop taking MMS, just take less. Go from 2 drops an hour of activated MMS to one drop an hour. Or if you are already take only one drop an hour, then take 1/2 drop and hour, or even 1/4 drop an hour. Do not cause yourself diarrhea if you can avoid it by taking less MMS. Pain, diarrhea, nausea and other discomforts cause loss of energy, which in turn causes slower healing and slower recovery. On the other hand try to increase the amount of drops you are taking until you are taking 3 drops an hour, but do not go over 3 drops an hour. Continue till you are well.

Portable 8 Hour Dose

Take a liter bottle, divide it into 8 equal parts. Mix 24 drops of MMS and 24 drops of 50% citric acid. Swirl or mix for about 20 seconds. Fill the bottle with water and you will have a 3 drops of MMS activated per line taken hourly.

MMS Protocols

Normal Dosage Defined

When following the suggestions below, keep this sentence in mind: Always activate one MMS drop with five drops of one of the food acids, either unfiltered vinegar, fresh lemon or lime juice, or citric acid solution (10% strength).

To make citric acid solution use a clean pint bottle with screw-on lid. Add 1 level tablespoon of citric acid powder and 9 tablespoons of water. Repeat that again if the bottle will hold it. Shake and store it in a capped jar. Refrigerate for longer life and to prevent thickening. Citric acid powder is available in most drug stores, enabling you to mix your own 10% liquid for storage.

In a cup or small glass always mix 5 drops of one of those food acids to each one drop of MMS. Swirl and wait at least 3 minutes, then add 1/3 to 2/3 to a full glass of water or thinned juice (but without any vitamin C) - then drink it. (You can expand the 3 minutes out to 10 minutes but no longer.) After adding the juice or water it is best if you drink immediately, but you can drink some, then wait as long as 30 minutes before drinking the second half without losing a lot too much of the beneficial ClO2 gas.

1. All methods for taking MMS begins with one or two drops. Never start with more than one or two drops. People who are very sick and sensitive should start with ½ drop (drink only half the glass of a one drop dose). Activate the MMS drops as given above.

2. If you do not produce nausea on the first dose, increase by one drop for the second dose. If you notice nausea reduce the amount of MMS for the next dose. It is important to understand that the chlorine dioxide that does all the good in your body only lasts a little more than one hour and then it is gone. Therefore to really do any good against the pathogens you are trying to kill, you need to continue the MMS continuously to the extent possible. Every two hours is usually OK. However, some people may prefer a morning and evening dose at first, then adding in a noon time dose while getting acclimated to the process. Some people want to ramp up faster than others, so proceed at your own speed.

Increase the number of drops taken every two hours. If you begin to feel nausea or diarrhea reduce the number of drops. Do not make yourself feel worse. Always take the maximum amount of MMS that you possibly can without getting nauseous or having diarrhea.

If you notice diarrhea, or even vomiting, that is not a bad sign. You are killing pathogens faster than your liver can process them for elimination. Therefore slow down the killing process. The body is simply throwing off poisons and cleaning itself out. Everyone says that they feel much better after the diarrhea. You do not have to take any medicine for the diarrhea. It will go away as fast as it came. It will not last. When the poison is gone, the diarrhea will be gone.

You must not continue to take so much MMS that it causes continued diarrhea or nausea. If diarrhea continues more than two days, keep reducing the dose and putting more hours between doses until there is no diarrhea.

During the Diarrhea stage watch for possible and unexpected parasites dropping into the commode. There are several types and varieties. Watch for small eggs which were going to hatch into parasites. If you see parasites you should not assume that this is the last of them. If you skip days of MMS treatment the parasites can reappear a month later. Avoid time gaps and keep a small amount of MMS circulating day and night to the extent you can tolerate. With parasites you will want to achieve complete clearance.

3. Continue to follow the procedure given in 2 above until you reach 12 drops taken every 2 or 3 hours - if possible - ALWAYS STAYING JUST UNDER THE NAUSEA BARRIER. Continue at three or more doses per day for at least one week and then reduce the drops to 4 to 6 drops a day for older people and 4 to 6 drops twice a week for younger people. Known as "maintenance" mode.

Once you have completed the step 3 above most of the viral, bacteria, mold, and yeast load will be gone from your body. Your body will be clean and cleared of the pathogens you picked up and hosted since childhood. You no longer have to worry about feeding the microorganism load. You can base your diet on nutrition, rather than not feeding the load.

Diabetes often goes away as inflammation of the pancreas diminishes. Your body will be able to easily absorb vitamins and minerals and many other nutrients it might have been missing up to this time. You should feel better as time goes by. Do not quit taking the MMS, Be sure to take vitamins and minerals and other nutrients that you know are good. MMS does not supply nutrients to your body so your normal program of nutrition should be maintained between doses or at night.

For Children the protocol is essentially the same. One should usually start at 1/2 drop. Just make a one drop drink and pour out 1/2 of the drink before giving it to the child. Then increase from 1 to 2 to 3 drops as given above, but do not go beyond 3 drops for each 25 pounds (11.4 kg) of body weight. With a baby start with 1/2 drop every 2 or 3 hours and stop when the baby is well.

If the baby or child should become nauseous wait an extra hour or two before giving another dose and also give a smaller dose. Give smaller doses until the baby or child can tolerate more, but do not stop giving doses until they are well. Children that are sick with the flu or other diseases should have 1/2 drop every hour during most of the day.

The Fundamentals for using MMS

Fundamental One:

Repeated small doses are more effective than large morning and evening doses. It has been demonstrated more than 1000 times that small doses administered often, up to once each hour, are more effective than large doses administered once or twice a day.

We now know that the chlorine dioxide chemical generated by MMS does not remain in the body more than one or two hours at most. The size of the dose does not seem to make a great deal of difference to the amount of time that MMS remains active in the body. That basically is because it does not matter if it is a large amount or small amount it still deteriorates into mostly just table salt in an hour or two.

So in reading the various methods of using MMS elsewhere on this web site, keep in mind - it is going to be much more effective to take MMS either each hour, or each two hours, and with smaller doses that will be equal to - or maybe larger than - one large dose.

If you are in the habit of taking larger MMS doses only in the morning and evening as was suggested in the past, MMS will still cleanse the body of microbes and pathogens. However, new research clearly reveals that a smaller-but-continuous circulation of ClO2 prevents regrouping and reproduction of pathogens, especially in situations where you are fighting a specific health issue - whether a cold or herpes or hepatitis.

After you are cleaned out a maintenance dose is still the same as always, 6 drops a day of MMS along with the citric or other acids required for activation. That's for older people and 6 drops twice a week for younger people, older people being over 60.

Fundamental Two:

Decrease the number of drops as needed if diarrhea or nausea occur, but do not stop taking MMS. Nausea and diarrhea are both good indicator signs that MMS is working. Diarrhea lasting for an hour or two is very good. To continue for longer periods can cause more harm than good. Always decrease the drops when these temporary barriers arise.

Fundamental Three:

Never take more than 3 drops and hour unless in a life threatening condition. In the case of life threatening situation use protocol 2000. See cancer

Fundamental Four:

Avoid all forms of Vitamin C for two hours before and after use of MMS. This is a temporary requirement necessary during these important weeks of increasing to the level of drops where you can be considered to be "Cleaned Out." If you are taking Vitamin C capsules marked as "12 hour" type, you will have to discontinue their use and only take capsules or tablets that do not indicate a timed action and take them only at night after MMS hours.

Fundamental Five:

Thoughtfully maintain a nutrition program adequate to maintain your immune system. MMS takes unwanted pathogens and parasites out of your body with great efficiency but it provides no nutritional minerals or vitamins. Maintain intake of friendly micro-organisms (acidophilus, and other flora). MMS itself does not kill intestinal friendly micro-organisms but forceful diarrhea can sometimes reduce their numbers. Similarly, maintain intake of minerals - especially calcium and magnesium.

Nutritional intake is critical to the immune system. Daily sun exposure will maintain your level of vitamin D. If you rarely see the sun you must maintain your vitamin D levels with supplements which are essential for maintaining the immune system. While MMS is the most potent germicidal agent on the planet, only the immune system produces healing and the maintenance of health.

MMS Protocols

Six proven ways to use MMS

1. Drink it. Swallow activated MMS with any amount of water or juice flavoring added. This is the most common method. Adding water or limited juice to the mix after the three minute wait enables you to drink the mixture. The amount of water matters very little provided that you drink it all - typically one half to a full glass of water. If you drink the entire amount you will get all of the MMS benefit. Diluted little or much it will still do the same cleansing within in your body.

After the three minute wait, when you add water or juice, no more chlorine dioxide is generated. It is locked into the water or juice. After drinking the mix with the water added, the ClO2 gas will circulate in the body for less than two hours as described above. Insignificant amounts of ClO2 are generated after the water is added, but not enough to consider.

You could repeat any MMS dose every two hours (or less) without harm provided you observe the temporary barriers created by diarrhea or nausea.

2. You can spray activated MMS on skin anywhere. It is effective against localized skin sores or diseases. The mixture must have a small amount of water added to make the liquid ready for spraying. It does not bleach hair and does not harm the skin. If you have open sores or cuts, it may cause sensations of burning but it promotes rapid germ-free closure of wounds.

3. MMS retention enemas are effective in cleansing intestinal walls. They also cause the ClO2 to be absorbed and mixed with the plasma of the blood - the blood liquid. MMS benefits are more available to more parts of the body more quickly when the ClO2 is carried in the plasma.

4. Hot tub baths with activated MMS in the water expose the entire skin surface to ClO2 ions. Add hot water continually while sitting in the tub. Skin pores open and the ClO2 ions pass deep below the skin and into muscles. Since blood is always present in muscles, the ClO2 ions merge into the plasma of the blood providing greater concentration of detoxifying action against parasites, yeast, fungus and other pathogens.

5. Some people briefly breath the ClO2 gas into the nose, head, and sinuses. DO NOT DEEPLY BREATH the ClO2 gas into the lungs because damage can happen to the lungs without you feeling it. Later you will find that you can almost not breath Sitting with your mouth or nose over a cup of activated 2 drop mixture (definitely no more than 2 drops), and with no water added, draw the odorous ClO2 gas into the nostrils or mouth. Approach this with caution. If it seems too strong move the cup further away or prepare a weaker mixture. The first time should be only two small breaths until you feel a tiny "bite."This has proven effective in killing germs in the sinuses that are often the cause of post-nasal drip. One or two brief nasal breathing session have been reported to eliminate post-nasal drip after all other medicines had failed to stop it.

Caution: If you have any history of asthma, use low doses and stop immediately if you have any sensation of an asthma attack. Never exceed the 4 drop maximum. This method is effective in situations where sinuses, vocal cords, or ear infections are retaining germs or pathogens.

Remember, it is the ClO2 Ion - the gas that you can smell - that is the germicidal agent. Use a 2 to 4 drop dose activated with 5 drops of citric acid or vinegar for each drop of MMS that you use. There's no need to add water since you will not be drinking it. Germs live and thrive in MUCUS and PHLEHM. The odor of ClO2 can kill them and prevent further production of mucus.

Some people report the feeling of catching a cold when using this method. Yes, there can be strong mucus films in your lungs from a cold you had a year ago known as Bio film. Bio film is also known in industry. Germs are sometimes encapsulated in the hardened but live mucus. The ClO2 gas weakens the mucus and the former cold germs escape. In this case, continue with internal 2 drop doses of activated MMS every hour (drink it), and continue deep breathing every four hours from the cup (Observe the limits and cautions above). The cold will soon vanish.

DO NOT EXCEED the 4 drop maximum and take only one or two breaths. You can always mix a second dose later if you want more time span. Bird cages and free-flying house birds should be kept in another room because of their sensitivity to various gases. HEED THESE CAUTIONS. You are responsible for using this strategy responsibly so avoid prolonged deep breathing of the ClO2 gas, always separated with deep breathing of normal air.

6. DMSO can sometimes be added to the MMS activated mix in special or life-threatening situations. Always test yourself first with a small DMSO spot on your arm. People who have a damaged or weakened liver should reduce the use of DMSO if any aching or pain is felt in the liver area. Put 1 or 2 drops of DMSO on your arm and rub it in. Wait for several hours. If there is no liver pain, you are probably safe in using DMSO.

One tablespoon of DMSO with two or more tablespoons of water can be taken internally by drinking it once or twice a day while fighting a severe disease. Normally use juice and dilute the DMSO much more. A 50-50 dilution will burn most people's throat. It's best to dilute DMSO with at least 2 parts water or juice to 1 part DMSO.

Caution One: DO NOT ATTEMPT any experimental intravenous injections in your home. There are health clinics that can administer such therapies. Seek qualified professionals who can take responsibility for proper dosage, administration, and predictable outcomes from any IV process. Health clinics may charge up to $100 per intravenous treatment. Intravenous provides about the same benefits as methods 4 and 5 above, but at a high cost.

Caution Two: If you choose to put activated MMS into a dehumidifier or room fogger, keep the MMS mixture at no more than 20 activated drops per gallon of water. (Must be activated in a cup with the three minute wait before dropping it into the water tank.) People have written asking about this. They want to use the humidifier because ClO2 is a powerful deodorizer and air purifier. Remove canaries and parrots from the room.

It is best not to sleep in the room where the humidifier is

fogging the room with ClO2 in the mix. Your lungs pick up the ClO2 gas (which is beneficial) just as readily as they pick up oxygen. While the ClO2 is received willingly by your lungs and red blood cells, you could unknowingly reduce oxygen intake and suffer harm. Remember this also if children are playing or sleeping in the same room. A limited amount of ClO2 in the air would be helpful for children and adults, but only if alert people are present and are knowledgeable about the nature of ClO2 as a germicidal agent.

It is equally effective to rid a closet or room of mold, odors, or germs if you set a 50 drop mix of activated MMS on a saucer in the middle of a closed room and let the ClO2 gas arise out of the liquid naturally. Do not add any water in this case. Do not exceed the 10 drop suggestion. It's more effective and safer to do several repeated room cleansing every hour than to release too much ClO2 at one time into a closed room. The odor does not linger and will not harm cushions, curtains, or lampshades. After 2 hours, the odor will have sacrificed itself and any room odors will be gone. If the normal small from shoes and clothes in a closet are still present, then a second ClO2 saucer or cup should be repeated.

ClO2 gas is a powerful deodorizer and germicidal agent. Drifting through the air, it will eventually kill all germs in the air and in furniture fabrics. After about two hours, the ClO2 gas disappears. It deteriorates into two molecules of water vapor. Activated MMS can restore lawn chairs thought to be ruined by skunk spray. Scrub the MMS mixture into car carpets, smelly shoes, and under arms. Will the whole house start to smell like a motel swimming pool? No. Not possible.

When using MMS as a room deodorizer or fungus eliminator, close the room doors and remove all pets and birds from the room for one or two hours.

Caution Three: Regarding Citric Acid: It is unusual to experience any nausea when starting MMS with a one drop dose. If you experience nausea after taking the first one-drop dose of MMS, it's rare, but you may be allergic to citric acid at the 10% solution strength. To quickly stop the nausea, wait ten minutes, then counter it with a teaspoon of baking soda in water if the nausea persists. Also eat an apple if you can keep it down. Wait overnight, then try a one-drop dose again, but use unfiltered and unpasteurized apple cider vinegar as the acid instead of citric acid.

It is very rare, but a few people are allergic to 10% citric acid in water, even though they may easily tolerate weak forms of it as in lemonade. The solution is to adopt unfiltered vinegar as the acid of choice because it is non-allergenic. Therefore try MMS again using unfiltered unpasteurized vinegar as the activating acid and slowly ramp upward in the number of drops.

The Advanced One to One Method

The protocols in this section refers to the one to one method or the 1:1 method for the use of MMS. This method has the same results as the original MMS method. The difference is the use of a 50% activator solution rather than a 10% solution (original protocol method) and the amount of time needed for activation. Please note the activation time is always 20 seconds when using this method.

The one to one method is a matter of preference and does not necessarily work better than the original protocols using a 10% solution. This advanced method is preferred by many for the small amount of time required for activation and because fewer drops need to be counted for preparation.

When in doubt always refer back to the following standard protocol for dosage amounts. This protocol will work for all circumstances.

Standard Advanced Protocol
The standard therapeutic dose is 3 drops of MMS activated. Use once per hour for an 8 hour period. Continue for three weeks or until cleansing events have ceased.

What are cleansing events?
Cleansing events are ways that the body releases un-metabolized waste and/or toxicity, which can happen in any combination of ways, including fever, swelling, inflammation, headaches, or other forms of aches and pain, diarrhea, or

vomiting. Generally, when these events occur our learned response is to take measures to stop the event. With the introduction of MMS people are learning that there's something worth looking forward to on the other side of that queasy feeling; energy, reduction in pain, healing, and best of all, health.

Sunburn and Burns

All burns should be sprayed with full strength MMS from a small spray bottle. DO NOT USE AN ACTIVATOR. If you do not have a spray bottle available apply MMS directly onto the burn, making sure the area is soaked.

Wait up to five minutes, but no longer before rinsing off. If you fail to rinse off, the burn will continue to hurt. On the other hand if you do rinse within 5 minutes the burn will heal in 1/4 the time normally required to heal. This includes all those terrible skin and flesh burns. The pain should stop immediately or reduce to almost zero within several minutes.

 Sunburns should be treated the same way. Spray the red area, wait 1 to 5 minutes, and rinse off. If the area is still sore, in about an hour spray the area again and wait 5 minutes before rinsing off. Remember, do not allow the MMS to stay in place. It must be rinsed off. Generally two doses will overcome most sunburns, but on rare occasions if the discomfort is not all gone you can use a third dose.

Note that MMS is alkaline and the burns need the alkalinity of the MMS to neutralize the acidity that resides in the burned areas. This is part of the reason why burns heal rapidly after the MMS applications.

Cancer Testing

Here is something your doctor will probably never tell you. There has been a medical test for cancer that is 99% effective for more than 25 years. It is more effective, less dangerous, and cheaper than all other medical cancer tests. It's called the AMAS' cancer test.

You do not have to go to a doctor; the test is available on the Internet. The cost is $165. The kit is free, you take a smear of your own blood, send it in and pay when the results are ready. The test is for specific cancer antibodies that will be present. Go to www.oncolabinc.com.

You can also get an idea about whether MMS will handle a cancer problem by evaluating the level of nausea you experience. You would start out at say one MMS drop or even 1/2 drop and observe that it does not make you nauseous. Then you begin to increase the drops twice a day once in the morning and once in the evening. That is if 1/2 drop does not make you nauseous in the morning, then in the evening or late afternoon try one full drop. Then the next morning take two drops and in the evening 3 drops.

Sooner or later the number of drops is going to make you nauseous. You then take a drop or two less the next dose for a time or two and continue to increase the drops. You are always looking for the nauseous point, taking less for a time or two and attempting to take more.

You will be able to know if it is going to help you if you can continue to pass the nausea point and increase the drops. What is happening is that when nausea hits, some of the cancer has been destroyed and it is now a poison that the body can clear out. Being able to clear out this poison is a part of it. The body can clear this poison out but it might generate some nausea in the process, or diarrhea or even vomiting. That's not bad.

The idea is that as the cancer is destroyed the body must clean out the poisons. As the cancer is destroyed the body can tolerate more and more drops. That's the indicator - is the body gradually being able to tolerate more and more drops? If you find that you can gradually increase the drops without getting nauseous it's an indicator that the body is doing the job.

In the case of cancer, you have to work at it. You start out slowly but increase quickly. At first you might just take the drops twice a day, but as you find you can do it twice a day without nausea, then increase to three times a day, and then four, and even as much as five times a day. Use Apples to overcome nausea. Use grated apples. Get a stainless steel grater. Do not buy the cheap tin grater. The grated metal cuts up the cells of the apple best. If a certain number of drops of MMS is making you nauseous, try at least two apples grated right after you take the MMS or just before you start getting nauseous. Always try the apples first, even two extra apples (4 altogether), but if you are still too sick, take as much as two teaspoons of baking soda in water.

What would indicate that you are not getting well is if the body got nauseous every time you take a dose no matter what amount of dose it is, and the body never seems to be able to increase the doses without nausea. But work at it. You can make it work. If you can take say two drops at a time without nausea and you get nausea when you go to three drops, you may have to tolerate the nausea for a short time, but if the nausea always occurs when you take three drops, it shows that you are not gaining on the cancer.

That can happen if the cancer is growing faster than the MMS is killing it. There is, however, always hope. One way would be instead of increasing the number of drops, increase the number of times that you take drops during the day. Read below. There are other actions that can help. Never, however, in any case stop taking the MMS.

So if there is an indication that one is not improving, then I suggest the following direction. Purchase some Indian Herb from Kathleen in Texas. It costs $60 a vial and that is plenty. Phone 806 647-1741 She has a thousand letters from people who have been helped. She and her father have been selling the Indian herb for over 60 years. When you get this herb use it with the MMS to get the best results. It comes with instructions.

The AMAS' cancer test listed above gives people a fantastic advantage. One can do a test, use the MMS for several weeks or a month and then do a second test to see how much improvement has taken place or to see if any improvement has happened at all.

Cancer Stages 1 to 3

This cancer procedure has been used enough times to convince us that it is the most successful so far for life threatening diseases. Normal flu and colds treatments do not need to be as intense as is described here.

We start new cancer patients that are very sick on 1 drop doses. So we use 1 and 1. That is a single drop dose and then wait an hour and then do the second drop dose. We do this in the morning, at noon and at night. That makes for 6 drops during a day for a very sick person. Some people might start at 2 and 2. Again that would be 2 drops and wait an hour and then two more drops. This would be done in the morning, at noon, and then in the evening before bed.

Depending upon how sick the person is, that determines the number of drops to use in the starting doses. A person who is in fairly good health could start at 6 and 6 drops doses.

However, no matter how many drops one starts with, if he does not notice any nausea the next day he should increase the number of drops by plus one. If the person started with 6 and 6 then the next day he would go to 7 and 7 three times during that day, and the day after it would be 8 and 8.

Anytime one notices nausea, always drop back a drop or two for up to a day before increasing the drops again. They should be increased slowly, carefully one drop a day until you are at 15 and 15. It may take a while to get to this point as the cancer should be almost cured by this time. Often the patient will get nauseous and you will have to drop back.

Advanced Stage Cancer

Begin with taking one drop of MMS each hour for at least 10 hours a day. The drop must be activated with one drop of the activator. You wait 20 seconds and then add 1/2 glass of water or juice and drink that. Do this every hour for 10 hours straight each day.

However, one drop is not enough, that is just to get you started. Once you determine that you can tolerate that one drop, go to two drops each hour. The one juice you must not use is orange juice. Stop the use of vitamin C while using this method.

You can increase up to 8 or even 10 drops of MMS each hour, however that is a lot, and most people will become nauseous and not tolerate that much until the cancer is completely gone. Place the activated mix in at least 3/4 glass of water - or more.

Enema

The MMS enema might be as effective as intravenous infusions since both methods dump MMS into the plasma of the blood and the red blood cell. This is the opinion of several biologists and scientists who have studied the enema method. Otherwise taking MMS by mouth generally delivers the chlorine dioxide to the red blood cells (only) from the stomach and intestines. The plasma will then have a tendency to carry the chlorine dioxide to areas that might not have the red blood cells visiting.

First clean yourself out with 32 ounces (one quart or 1000 ml approximately) of clean water. You can add a tablespoon of salt, or 1/2 cup of aloe vera juice, or other items recommended by nutritionists, but do not use coffee. Do the cleaning action two or three times. Put 32 ounces in and leave it as long as you can while exercising or massaging your stomach, and then let it out.

Then insert the activated MMS in a small amount of water of about 4 ounces. Use the same amount and the same procedure as if taking the MMS by mouth. Just as the protocol says, increase 1 or 2 drops of activated MMS each time. Do as many as 2 enemas a day. Try to keep the MMS in place and allow the colon walls to absorb the entire amount. Keep it up as if you were taking it by mouth. It will be more effective this way. Reduce the amount of MMS if you get diarrhea or nausea.

If you have a catheter it may work better, though not absolutely required. One then very carefully works the catheter into the colon so that the liquid is delivered a little over one foot inside.

Flu

You can use MMS both as a preventative and as a remedy to overcome Swine Flu. The method is to take MMS hourly.

1. In a clean dry glass mix 1 drop of MMS with 1 drop MMS Activator. Swirl and wait 20 seconds for activation.

2. .Add ½ glass of water or juice that does not have added ascorbic acid or vitamin C (Vitamin C prevents proper functions of this solution). Drink this whole amount as quickly as possible.

3. If you felt absolutely no change during this first hour, go ahead and go to 2 drops on the second hour and so on. Over time increase to a maximum of 6 drops MMS with 6 drops of the activator.

Keep in mind that most people will not go over 3 or 4 drops an hour before they begin to feel added nausea. Upon any sensation of nausea, reduce the number of drops by at least one drop. Nausea occurs when MMS is killing germs and viruses faster than your elimination system can handle the debris.

4. Continue taking MMS each hour for 12 hours. The flu should be gone by the end of 12 hours. Do not stop taking the MMS until you are sure you have recovered. If you still feel flu symptoms the next day be sure to continue on the same hourly doses. Children can have the same treatment except be extra cautious to prevent nausea or sick feeling. Do this by using smaller doses. Increase by 1/2 drop each time and never go above 3 drops an hour.

5. Continue to take a six drop dose twice a day for the next week or two.

6. To prevent the flu and maintain you immune system in top condition take one 6 drop dose of MMS every day for adults and children should take a dose each day depending upon their age or size. Use 1 drop for each 25 pounds of body weight, and 1 drop for babies.

Fungus

It would have been simpler if MMS had been able to handle everything in the disease world, but there seems to be a fungus that MMS simply does not touch. In fact, MMS seems to feed the fungus. This fungus can occur in the feet, or hands or most any other place in the body.

It is not athlete's feet, it is much worse. All the athletes foot sprays and powders do not touch it. It can occur on the skin, and it seems to be much worse than any other skin infection. It itches and burns terribly and it appears to be under the skin as well as on the skin. It makes the skin slightly puff up, and it looks bad and it gets worse.

The name of this fungus has not been identified. It can last for years. I do not know if it has ever been fatal, but it seems to be very bad and sometimes it can get into the mouth and gums and cause much suffering. It also happens on the head or scalp where it causes havoc.

This particular fungus reacts to MMS with a stinging burning pain. It will almost always be worse after being treated with MMS. Your feet can be so bad that you cannot walk. This is the only way to identify it that I know of.
Luckily this particular fungus is rather rare. It does not happen in very many people. However, I have included it here as I do not know any other treatment than what I am about to tell of.

So if you have athlete's feet that will not go away, or gum disease that MMS will not cure in less than one week, or skin disease that just cannot be treated successfully, then this is what to do, and do not worry, it will not do any harm.

Use Bentonite clay, in France it is called Montmorillonite. Mix this clay 50-50 with Vaseline (petroleum jelly). Then smear it on the various areas. If your problem is in the feet, smear it on the feet and cover it with thick socks. If it is on the skin, smear it on the entire area of the infection.

If you do not use the Vaseline it will not work very well. Vaseline makes it contact the skin and tissues and does something that makes it work much better. Do not use the Vaseline in your mouth. Just brush your teeth with the Bentonite Clay powder just like using any particular tooth powder. Brush them gently, but three or four times a day.

The fungus infection should clear up in about one week. However, I would keep a light coating on for a month or so. This treatment has helped a number of people so far.

One more thing: There is always the possibility of getting a similar fungus infection inside the body. In that case, use the same clay inside the body by taking it by mouth. Start with 1 teaspoon of clay in ½ glass of water or juice and in several days work up to 2 tablespoon full's (rounded) a day.

Molecular silver solution has also produced very good results. Some people use this two hours after MMS doses to speed or supplement the MMS germicidal benefits. Molecular silver is superior to most colloidal silver because it is manufactured with high voltages and is much higher in germicidal action.

HIV and Aids

Take 3 drops of activated MMS in juice or water for at least 8 hours straight every day for 3 weeks. Only those people who are very sick need to start out at less than 3 drops and hour. Use 3 drops of MMS and 3 drops of MMS Activator, wait 20 seconds and add 1/4 to 1/2 glass of juice or water and drink. Do not use orange juice, most other juices are OK. If you notice nausea, or vomiting, or diarrhea, stop until the problem is gone, and then continue with less MMS for a few hours. But return to 3 drops an hour as soon as you can.

If bad nausea persists take as little as 1/4 drop and hour. It's OK to stop until nausea is gone, but a small amount of nausea may continue for some time. Do not let a tiny bit of nausea stop you. Only stop if it gets to be irritating. NORMALLY VERY LITTLE NAUSEA OR DIARRHEA IS NOTICED, BUT IT DOES HAPPEN. If you have to go to 1/4 or 1/2 drop for a long time to prevent nausea that is OK but you should then extend your protocol an extra week.

The nausea is caused by killing pathogens as the pathogens dump poison into the system when they die. A normal healthy person notices absolutely nothing from taking a great deal more than 3 drops an hour. The more health problems the more likely you will be to notice nausea. Just handle it as given above and you will be OK.

Normally HIV positive people have what is called opportunity diseases that take over or get started because of the distressed immune system. Evidently the first thing MMS does is to go after those diseases. It provides ammunition to the immune system. The immune system then runs out and kills the pathogens throughout the body.

Hourly doses are required is because HIV is a virus. I know there are theories that HIV does not exist and that AIDS does not come from HIV. And the fact is about 50% of the people who have AIDS never were diagnosed with HIV. Fortunately, MMS does not care one bit either way. MMS kills viruses in a different way than bacteria. It prevents the growth of viruses by preventing the formation of the special virus proteins.

However, it has been demonstrated that this takes longer than just blowing a hole in the side of the bacteria. It evidently takes more than 1 or 2 hours. How much longer I am not sure, but the 3 drops hourly for 8 hours per day for 3 weeks seems to work.

Intravenous

Needed Supplies:

1 - 250 ml bag of saline or glucose solution with the standard needle and tubing for IV. We use saline solution usually unless we expect a drop in blood pressure, in which case the glucose seems to keep the blood pressure up. It has been suggested by a doctor that it is best to use no more than 250 ml solutions for 1 hour drips. He mentioned that it can cause water on the lungs in larger doses. Tie the bag in place and get set to use it.

1- bottle MMS Advanced

1- bottle MMS Advanced Activator

MMS Protocols

1- hypodermic syringe

1- experienced nurse or Doctor

Use a dry clean glass. Do not worry about disinfecting the glass as the MMS will do that. Use 1 drop MMS and 1 drop MMS Activator, shake to mix, wait 20 seconds, using the syringe remove several (ml) from the IV bag, add the solution from the bag into a glass and mix with the MMS. Suck the solution mixed with the MMS back into the syringe and squirt it back into the IV bag. Shake the bag a bit to mix it. It's ready to use.

Set the drip for approximately one hour. The herxheimer reaction, if there is one, will probably start in 1 to 2 hours. Keep the patient warm. Normally it lasts 2 hours or less.

Do the same MMS IV dose the second day or twice in one day, morning and evening. Continue until there is no herxheimer reaction and then go to the next higher dose. Continue at that dose until there is no reaction at that level and then go to the next higher dose again until you have reached 22 drops of MMS and 22 drops of MMS Advanced Activator. Continue at this level until the patient reports that he is better or cured.

Of course, observe the patient and make sure that reactions are herxheimer reactions and not other problems. Do not make the patient sick. Reduce the number of drops used if the patient continues to experience chills, or headaches, or nausea, or diarrhea. Do not stop, just drop back in the number of drops being used until the patient can tolerate the condition without discomfort.

About the pain of IV infusions: Normally there should be no pain involved in IV infusions. A number of doctors have mentioned to me that they expected pain because of the citric acid used. But that does not make a lot of sense. For example in a large dose of MMS, like 15 drops plus 75 drops of citric acid solution when mixed you create one teaspoon of MMS at a pH (acid/alkaline balance) of 4.8. That is not a strong acid. And when that is added to 250 ml of IV solution you are not going to change the pH balance by enough to record unless you have a very delicate instrument. I guarantee not enough for the inside of your veins to feel. If you use pH test paper I guarantee that you will not be able to tell the difference in the pH balance between before adding the MMS and after adding the MMS.

The pain is either created by poorly inserting the needle or by using the veins in the hands. I am sorry I do not know why the hand causes the pain, but it seems to cause it. It is some sort of neurological response as opposed to the feeling of acid against the vein walls. When the needle is properly inserted in the arm instead of the hand, there is almost never any pain. If the pain was coming from the blood vessel, it would only hurt right at the vessel, but that is not the case. The whole arm hurts and that has to be some sort of nervous reaction.

The needle must penetrate the skin and the vein in the same place. If the needle slides along the vein before it penetrates there will be pain and usually inflammation. So it sort of gets to be a scientific art. You got to get it right to prevent the pain. Just a tiny bit of MMS in the skin or tissue and you have the pain and that multiplies.

Life Threatening

Regarding life-threatening situations the goal would be to more quickly get MMS circulating in the blood while trying to stay under the nausea barrier.

One way to achieve this is by adding DMSO to the activated MMS so that it can act as a carrier for sending MMS directly into the skin and muscles of the body and thus into the blood of the body.

Experience and testing has proved that DMSO is carried directly to any cancer in the body and it then penetrates the cells of the cancer. This is not theory, but has been proved through testing. In this case when the DMSO is carrying MMS the theory is that it will carry the MMS into the cancerous cells killing the virus that causes the cell to be cancerous.

Do This Test First

A few people are allergic to DMSO or have very weak livers and can have bad problems with DMSO. Wash your arm carefully and dry it. Then add one drop of DMSO to one spot on your arm and rub it in. Give it about 15 minutes to soak in and then wait several hours. If there is no pain in your liver area you are probably safe in using DMSO which will be the case in 99 people out of 100. To be safe, wait another 24 hours to make sure there is no reaction to the DMSO.

In this case, I found by testing that after three minutes of stirring the MMS and the acid as is normal, the DMSO should be added to the mix immediately without further delay. Otherwise much of the power of the MMS is wasted or lost. I suggest stirring the activated MMS with the DMSO for only 15 seconds. Then immediately rub it onto a large area of the body like a leg or arm. This may get as much as 5 times more MMS through the skin and into the blood stream. And of course, using a larger area of the body can also get more MMS into the blood stream.

Taking MMS as described below is an accelerated skin treatment technique that pushes MMS into the plasma of the blood in addition to the normal oral doses of MMS. Exact steps follow:

1. Prepare a dose of MMS by activating 10 drops of MMS with 10 drops of MMS Activator. Swirl or stir it for several seconds and wait for 20 seconds.

2. Add one teaspoon of DMSO and stir it for about 15 seconds, no longer.

3. Immediately rub it on to a leg or arm or belly. Do not wait any time at all as the solution is quickly losing strength as time passes. For example, a three minute wait would be too long.

You can use a plastic sack with your hand inside to rub the solution onto your body, or you can just use a bare hand or hands. If you noticing any burning sensation you can add a teaspoon full of water to the area that is burning and rub it in. Keep that up until there is no more burning. You can rub olive oil and aloe vera juice on the skin after the application. Use a different part of the body each time you apply the MMS/DMSO.

4. Do this once every other hour the first day, and once every

hour the second day, and third day, and then quit for 4 days and start the same thing the next week, but never stop taking the MMS by mouth.

DMSO is a well-known carrier substance used widely by doctors since 1955 as a way to carry medications directly into the skin. It is available in drugstores in most states, and also on the Internet.

Maintenance Dose

MMS maintenance doses and can reduce your risk by a very large amount, maybe as much as 95%. MMS supercharges your immune system by providing a chemical that the immune systems needs to kill various pathogens.

Assuming you have "graduated" from the body cleansing process in which you took more and more drops of activated MMS (morning and night) up to a maximum of 15 drops morning and night - holding that level for five to seven days, then in most cases you are probably quite well cleared of body toxins, poisons, heavy metals, yeast, and fungus.

Having achieved that 15 drop level - and understanding that you may or may not get to that level in one month due to temporary diarrhea or temporary nausea barriers, after graduation, you should drop back to a lower maintenance dosage.
One example might be one eight-drop dose on Monday and Thursday mornings at 6 am, then breakfast at 8 am, thus achieving maximum Cl02 benefits.

Another example might be taking a six-drop dose every morning, except Saturday and Sunday.

One factor to consider is that MMS doses at almost any level are one of the best cancer preventatives. It seems certain now that cancer is caused by a morphing microbe that gets inside a normal cell after circulating by blood to its resting place. That microbe would never find a hosting place among your cells if even a little MMS was circulating as often as possible. A small amount taken frequently might prevent the formation and development of cancer.

Adjust the maintenance dose according to your own needs.

Malaria

Malaria victims are divided into two groups - adults and children. Many hundreds of children have been given MMS doses according to 3 drops for each 25 pounds (11.4 kg) of body weight.

Adults are first given 15 drops. Every drop of MMS is always activated with 1 drop of MMS Activator. Once the activator is added, one must wait 20 seconds before adding 1/2 glass of water or apple or pineapple juice. The drink is immediately consumed.

One must wait only one hour and then the malaria victim is given a second dose of the same size. All symptoms of malaria should be gone after 4 hours beyond the second dose.

If all the symptoms are not gone on the following morning or even later that evening a third dose of 15 drops of MMS should be give to adults and made in the same way as given above. A third dose for the child who has not become well should simply be double the first dose.

One must then wait only an hour. Then the victim should be given the fourth dose the same as above using 15 drops for an adult and double dose for a child. The patient should be malaria free within 12 hours. Ninety-nine percent of the malaria victims will be handled at this point.

However, with any malaria victim that continues to be sick, they should continue to receive doses at 4 hour intervals (3 times a day) but reduce the number of drops in a dose if the patient is nauseous. Continue as long as the patient is sick, but continue with doses as high as possible that do not make the patient nauseous.

These suggestions are based on the personal treatment of thousands of people who had failed to eliminate malaria from their bodies using all other known means. Many were dying or near to death.

Mouth and Gums

Cleansing Mouthwash:
Mouth and gum diseases respond promptly to MMS. Just make up a 10 drops dose of MMS. Take 10 drops of MMS and add 10 drops of Activator, wait 20 seconds and then add about 1/2 glass of water (4 ounces).

Use a soft tooth brush and pour the liquid onto the brush and brush your teeth and gums very well. Be gentle at first. Do this 3 or 4 times a day for the first three or four days. Then do it once a day.

Use the extra solution to rinse and gargle your mouth. Do this slowly so that some of the Cl02 gas has time to simmer out of the liquid. The invisible Cl02 gas will kill all the germs and bacteria in your mouth without harming sensitive gums or sore places on the tongue. Then for a few weeks brush your teeth at least once a day with the MMS solution.

Your mouth should be in much better condition after one week, but it will continue to improve for several weeks before it gets to the condition of being a lot healthier than ever before. You can then cut back to two or three times a week.

Emergency Toothache Options:
There are many reports of people whose toothaches were stopped completely within a few minutes of holding activated MMS in the mouth for two minutes. This would be one of those situations where you could not get scheduled for dental work and you have no choice but to clinch down on cloves to mask the pain - which might mean days or weeks while you wait for an opening on the dentist's waiting list.

However, after one or two MMS treatments, the tooth ache might not reappear for 12 to 24 hours. The reason for tooth-pain is usually that bacteria has found a home deep in a tooth cavity and bacteria are feeding on nutrients near or touching the nerve. By holding even a low MMS mixture in your mouth and brushing heavily on the tooth surface where the cavity might be, the odor of Cl02 can be forced into the tooth far enough that the bacteria "smell it," stop nibbling, and die near the nerve. The tooth will not cause any more pain until more food is pressed into the crevice and new bacteria begin feeding again.

This procedure can be executed with a low dosage like this: one MMS drop in a small cup with one drop of the MMS Advanced Activator. After 20 seconds, add 1 or 2 table spoons of water and stir it with a toothbrush. Your toothbrush is now nicely sterilized. Stir the mixture onto the brush, carry it into your mouth, and brush the tooth or teeth where the pain is felt. Carry more MMS into your mouth and repeat for two minutes or more.

Pressure-sensitive Tooth:
It should be noted that if your tooth is pressure sensitive - meaning that when you bite down on it then pain is felt, this usually indicates a pocket of infection forming under the tooth. In this case, mere brushing is futile but you have a powerful option for reducing and eliminating the infected tooth. Do it quickly.

Immediately start taking your normal MMS doses MORE OFTEN. Get the MMS and ClO2 circulating as soon as possible. For example, if you were normally taking 8 drop doses morning and night, step it up - take your doses every two hours - for two days until at least, or until the tooth pressure-pain disappears. The infection will in most cases be eliminated without a terrifying root canal procedure. You will avoid strong antibiotics that dentists give to kill the infection. You will avoid further dental work to "save the tooth." This suggestion is based on actual experiences and user reports.

Candida and Bad Breath:
While your one-drop mixture lasts, if you have any white candida film on your tongue, brush your tongue.

While in there with brush in hand, if you have bad breath, brush the extreme back of the tongue where sulfur dioxide is produced by some types of bacteria. One clinic has a patented tongue brush and a special MMS-like fluid that quenches the bad-breath bacteria. But in your case you already have MMS which produces Cl02 gas, and a tooth brush already in your mouth, so shove the brush back to the gagging point and clean the back of your tongue.

Brighten Your Teeth:
There is misinformation about MMS causing teeth to be darkened. This is not the case. MMS has a gradual whitening effect on teeth. Years of tartar and accumulated colorings are slowly lifted away.

Plaque Buildup:
Questions arise regarding whether MMS can remove plaque without dental assistance. No, it might take years of twice daily brushing with MMS to diminish thickened plaque that developed over the years. It's probably better to pay a dental assistant to remove plaque using the tools they have. THEN AFTER THAT, you can prevent or diminish greatly the formation of new plaque. Dental assistants are usually trained to tell you that plaque is normal, that everyone needs to come back four times a year for plaque removal. You may be told that there is SLIME in everybody's mouth and during the night it lays down additional film whether you brush or not.

Unless your genetics cause you to produce SLIME IN ABUNDANCE, a night and morning MMS mouthwash and light brushing will leave you with a germ free mouth. The slime will evaporate through the night, having no bacterial assistance to create layers of tartar and plaque.

Nose, Sinus, Ear, Bronchial Congestion

This MMS protocol comes with CAUTIONS but it is very effective in eliminating post-nasal drip, sinus infections, ear infections, head colds, sore throats, wheezing, bronchitis, and germs that live in nose or sinus mucus. Even inner ear infections are reported to benefit from this treatment. But, there are CAUTIONS.

You will be inhaling small amounts of the ClO2 gas from a cup into your nose or mouth. OBSERVE THE CAUTIONS LISTED BELOW.

Do not drink the mixture in this protocol because no water is added to the activated MMS in this instance. Do not exceed a 2 or 3 drop mixture. Remember, it is the ClO2 gas generated by MMS that is the entire germ-killing benefit. Unlike the MMS mixture that you drink, this method of nose-inhaling the pure ClO2 gas probably provides the quickest and most germicidal way to move the gas quickly to places in the head and sinuses where it can easily find germs and kill them.

However, a severe warning is stated - DO NOT OVERDOSE. DO NOT DEEP BREATH THE ClO2 gas into your lungs for any length of time. Your lungs can rapidly absorb the ClO2 gas just as easily as oxygen, causing unexpected depletion of oxygen. Take breaks and breath normal air periodically while doing this procedure. This warning will be repeated several times. IF YOU OVERDOSE AND DEEP BREATH YOU MAY DAMAGE YOUR LUNGS.

Prepare 2 to 3 drops of MMS with 2 to 3 drops of MMS Activator in equal parts. Do this in a small cup. Do not add water or anything else. DO NOT DRINK THIS MIXTURE.

Almost immediately you will smell the ClO2 gas. Holding the cup under your nose pull in the gas slowly with the goal of letting it pause to circulate in the nose and sinus cavities. It will naturally flow also down through the throat and vocal cords to some extent. Breath it into the nose very slowly so that it lingers a bit in all places it can go. Hold that breath for a few seconds. The ClO2 odor will even be wafted out into the estuation tubes and sometimes out to the inner ears.

After every four slow inhaling actions, move the cup away and take in breaths of normal air.

REASON FOR CAUTION. You are moving pure ClO2 gas directly into the body. Your red blood cells absorb it as readily as oxygen. Therefore you will be temporarily diminishing the amount of oxygen available to your body.

DO NOT USE THIS METHOD if you suffer from Angina, or if you are dependent on supplemental oxygen for breathing, or if you have shortness of breath, or if you have been using MMS internally (drinking it with water) above the 10 drop level during the past two hours.

When you drink MMS doses, the ClO2 is generated slowly. Red blood cells pick up normal oxygen from the lungs, but perhaps 20% of them accidentally do not pick up oxygen. A bit later the blood passes around the stomach lining and the 20% of red blood cells that lacked oxygen pick up ClO2 because it looks like oxygen to the red blood cells. So in normal MMS use (when drinking it), oxygen is still available to the body just as it is normally and the amount of ClO2 absorption is self-limiting because 80% (for example) of the red blood cells are supplying oxygen to the body as they normally do.

In summary: when breathing ClO2 as a gas freshly produced in a small cup, as it is held for a few seconds in the sinuses, nose, and vocal cords, it has immediate germicidal effects as it encounters germs and pathogens along the way, thus reducing the generation of mucus and phlegm.

Cold germs and flu viruses live in the mucus produced by the body in reaction to the germs or viruses. Lungs and sinuses begin to weep, generating sticky fluids in the sinuses, lungs, and bronchioles. Germs then continue to reproduce and travel further in that mucus - unless the germs are killed by an outside agent such as MMS.

It is critical that no one should have a bad experience with MMS. So as a further caution, think about the results if you foolishly overdose with this protocol:

1. Instead of 15% of the red blood cells carrying ClO2 throughout the body, you could crowd out necessary oxygen if 25% or 30% of your red blood cells pickup ClO2 instead of oxygen. Therefore after 4 or 5 deep slow inhalations from the

cup, take a break so that your oxygen supply is not diminished to your brain or body.

2. Since this method supplies pure ClO2 directly into the body, it will be circulated quickly throughout the body resulting in RAPID KILLING of pathogens throughout the body - possibly resulting in severe and sudden nausea as debris from rapid detoxification is spilled too rapidly into the blood.

3. Lung tissues can be burned or damaged without you being aware that you are overdosing.

4. You could pass out from thoughtless deep breathing. The odor of the ClO2 gas is quite easy to breath. Unlike the bad taste of activated MMS in water, the odor of MMS is not bad enough to prevent overdosing. In fact you may think that nothing is happening and could be tricked into thinking that stronger doses or deeper breathing can be tolerated. BE THOUGHTFUL and DO NOT OVERDOSE.

5. Placing activated MMS into a humidifier would keep a continuous flow of odorless ClO2 in the air for one to two hours, but there is no need to do this because of the danger of sleeping or living in a depleted oxygen state. The room has plenty of oxygen but your lungs adsorb the ClO2 as readily as the oxygen which is a dangerous situation if prolonged for any length of time.

6. Remove pets and birds from the room if you are using the ClO2 gas as a way to remove fungus or mold from a room. Close the doors during the hour of ClO2 room cleansing. For purification of a room, place a 10 to 20 drop mixture of

activated MMS in a saucer or cup in the middle of the room, then close and leave it for one hour. The ClO2 fumes will emerge slowly and fill the room over time.

Skin Care

The use of MMS on the skin can be a very important. It destroys almost every kind of skin disorder known, and causes burns, and wounds of all kinds to heal often in less that 1/2 the ordinary time.

So here are the basics regarding skin treatment with MMS. I have completed more than 6 months spraying my body every day with a very strong solution of Activated MMS.

I sprayed in many places on my body to see the results on heavy weather beaten skin to the most tender white skin available. I usually sprayed several times a day. I sprayed on my face most days as well, and often rubbed around my eyes so that the rubbing would allow a tiny amount of MMS to leak into the eye itself.

There were places where I did not spray to show the difference between treated areas and untreated areas over a period of six months. The results were this: After more than six months, there was no difference between the areas sprayed and the areas not sprayed. There was no skin discoloring, nor any change in the texture, nor any other kind of change including on my face.

During the six months, there were times when small wounds or cuts happened. These I always sprayed and they disappeared in a day or two.

MMS does not affect normal body cells. It does not have the power. It only kills anaerobic microorganisms on the skin or in the body. Tests have been made with similar sprays at this strength and less in slaughter yards on dead animal skins and dead chicken skins and all anaerobic microorganisms are always dead.

Use MMS for healing sores, burns, wounds, psoriasis, eczema, cancer, ringworm, acne, rashes, staph infections, athletes feet, and a hundred other problems of the skin. In order to do this follow these instructions: Obtain a 2 ounce mist spray bottle. Most drug stores sell empty spray bottles.

Add 20 drops of MMS in the bottle then and 20 drops of MMS Activator and swirl to mix, wait 20 seconds and then fill the bottle with water. You now have a spray solution that is equivalent to 40 drops in 1/2 glass of water in strength. This solution stays fresh for about 3 days. The reason it stays fresh for that long is that of the strength. Once it is diluted in the body it rapidly disintegrates. Or on the skin, it disintegrates as it dries.

Once you have made your solution, you should spray any sore about once an hour or every two or three hours all day long. Allow the solution to dry on the sore. In case of a rash, spray it on the entire rash. Rinse off with clean water in the evening before bed, dry, and re-spray before going to bed. In case of babies under 2 years old I would suggest that you dilute the solution at least twice or start out with only 5 drops of MMS instead of 20.

The MMS in the spray bottle will seldom ever cause stinging or burning or pain, but it can happen. If it does, pour out 1/2 of the liquid in the bottle and fill it with water thus diluting by 50%. If it still stings, do the same thing thus diluting it again. Continue this dilution until it does not sting.

In one person out of a thousand persons with skin problems, the MMS may sting badly and the problem will get worse. If this happens it is probably a condition that you have had for a long time. This is very rare, but it does happen. Do not feel badly, there is a cure. Look in the section for fungus.

Taste

Using the capsule Method

This method will enable you to take MMS without the bad taste.

You can buy empty vegetable gel capsules at most health food stores. The capsules go by sizes called "SIZE ZERO" and "SIZE ONE." Size zero holds 250 mg of powder or tiny granules – untamped.

What you will need:
Empty vegetable gel capsules as noted.
Clean bulb Eyedropper

Prepare the capsule: If you are going to take a 4 drop dose, put 4 drops of MMS in the corner of a clean dry glass, then drop 4 drops of Activator on the MMS drops and shake the glass while tipped and wait 20 seconds.

Now take a clean eye dropper and pick up the drops from the glass and put them into the large half of a gel capsule and immediately put on the other half as a lid and then wash the capsule down with a 1/2 glass of water or more.

Follow this same procedure with any amount of drops up to 5 drops of MMS and 5 drops of MMS Activator. The size 0 capsules will actually hold about 13 drops total. For a larger dose use two capsules.

Tub Bathing

Bathing in MMS water enables cleansing of pathogens that are on the skin surface or just under it. Cleansing at these outer levels seems to avoid overloading the internal elimination systems. Pathogens killed near the skin surface more-often move outward through the skin and float away. Do continue with normal MMS oral doses.

1. WIPE OUT THE TUB. Otherwise the MMS ClO2 gas in the water will go to work on any soap scum and bathtub-ring, reducing or neutralizing the Cl02 available to the body. By the second bath, the tub will be clean due to the MMS cleansing action. Put no soap or other chemicals in the water. Adding more water does not weaken the CL02 that is being generated. Some people add 1/4 cup DMSO. (Not required but it may assist deeper penetration of the Cl02 gas.)

2. ACTIVATE MMS IN A CUP OR GLASS before adding to

the tub water. Place 30 drops of MMS in a cup. Add 30 drops of the MMS Activator. Plan for a 20 to 30 minute tub sitting. If you have open skin sores or severe body wounds consider reducing the MMS to 20 drops mixed with 20 drops of the MMS Activator so that sensations of heat or burning will be reduced. Open sores usually heal quickly due to the disinfecting action of MMS.

3. MIX THE MMS WITH THE ACTIVATOR AND SWIRL IN A CUP Wait 20 seconds. While waiting, draw 5 to 8 inches of hot water for bathing. Do not add soap, perfume, or shampoo. The amount of water does not matter. It is good to drink a separate 6 or 8 drop dose as well.

4. ADD THE ACTIVATED MMS into the tub water. Stir it. Almost immediately all germs in the water will be eradicated. Water does not reduce the amount of ClO2 gas that is being produced. Tub half full or very full does not matter because the same amount of Cl02 gas will be produced by the activated MMS.

5. LAY IN THE TUB. One side, then the other. Splash water onto the entire body - arms, neck, hair, face - all over. If a history of cold sores, then wipe tub water on the lips and nose repeatedly and wherever they were once visible. If water splashes in the eyes, just wipe it away. MMS does not harm eyes - unlike shampoo. With a cup pour tub water onto the scalp.

6. ADD MORE HOT WATER. Heat opens the pores and MMS penetrates into the muscles. Massage the scalp with tub water. By the 3rd bath, skin moles may begin to crumble.

7. WIPE AWAY TUB DEBRIS when finished.

Viruses

Viruses are a thousand times smaller than bacteria and thus are not killed in the same way. Bacteria are killed by an explosive oxidation reaction, whereas viruses are killed by keeping a virus from forming over a period of time. MMS prevents the protein of the virus from growing into its final configuration and thus they die.

Where viral diseases are present, you must keep MMS present in the body for an extended period so that viruses cannot continue to build their special proteins.

The various protocols take this into consideration. For viral infections, normally the chlorine dioxide needs to be continuously present in low-dose amounts for at least 12 hours, and sometimes even longer. This is in contrast with bacterial infections where a large dose of MMS in the morning, noon, and evening will be effective in a fast kill of bacteria.

We know for certain that activated MMS (chlorine dioxide) only remains present in the body for about 1 hour. That means you must take a small amount of MMS every hour for an extended period to keep the viruses from forming, and thus they die by never reaching maturity.

Take as much MMS as you can handle without getting sicker or nauseous. Start out with one drop, and in an hour take two drops, then three drops at the third hour. Keep increasing, but drop back a drop or two if you notice nausea.

It's OK to sleep without taking MMS through the night but begin again the next day until you are well.

Questions and Answers

This section will answer most of your questions about MMS regarding the many different health conditions. Please keep in mind that the protocols in the answer to each question here refers to the original protocol using a 10% solution for activation and a 3 minute activation time. You may alter the original protocol and use the advanced one to one protocol by substituting a 50% solution for activation and shortening the activation time to 20 seconds.

The text in this section has not been edited in order to preserve the integrity of the questions asked. Likewise the answers in this section have not been edited to preserve original content. All answers were given by Jim.

The questions here are categorized by health condition.

Aerobic

How does MMS kill the bacteria?

Q: If the MMS kills bacteria, how does it deal with the body's natural bacteria which consists of 80% good and 20% bad? I know you state that it leaves healthy cells and kills the harmful ones, but can it differentiate between bacteria and leave the body's natural bacteria (good and bad) alone? If all the bacteria is destroyed are you promoting a pro-biotic?

A: Good bacteria in the body are known as aerobic bacteria (that means that they use oxygen). Disease causing bacteria are Anaerobic (that means they do not use oxygen). You might suppose then, that there is some sort of difference between them and that is true, there is a difference. Guess what, the unique qualities of the MMS ion (chlorine dioxide) allows it to see the difference between the two different bacteria, and thus it only destroys the anaerobic bacteria (that's the disease causing bacteria). This is also controlled by the white blood cells in the immune system which have the ability to use chlorine dioxide against the diseases.

Allergies

Can you help me with some suggestions about dosages?

Q: I would be grateful for your suggestions concerning dosages/usage of the MMS and the water combo package with the Prill beads & balls for maximum benefit: Person #1 is recovering from breast cancer, is a smoker, and has undergone chemo: Person #2 is paraplegic with chronic bladder/kidney infections [also ordered colloidal silver for him], asthma and allergies, anxiety attacks and chronic depression, suspected add or onset of bipolar disorder Person #3 is type 2 diabetic, high blood pressure, high cholesterol, degenerative arthritic condition, chronic obesity.

A: All these people you mention should follow the standard protocol for MMS. Start with two drops MMS, add ten drops of lemon or lime or citric acid solution as described in my book, mix, allow to set three minutes, add 1/2 glass or water and drink. Go the three drops, then to four, four and then to 5. each time always using the correct amount of lemon or lime juice or citric acid solution. If nausea occurs, take a drop or two less the next time. Then, keep increasing the drops until you have reached 15 drops a day for 5 or 6 days then increase to three 15 drop doses a day until the problem is gone. Do not remain at three 15 drop doses a day for longer than 2 months. Reduce the amount as soon as possible. Then decrease to 4 to 6 drops a day for maintenance.

How should I handle my cat allergy?

Q: I am allergic to cats, in Panama I caught some kind of fungus or mold or something in my lungs. Maybe because of my allergy, my infection has been worst. I am up to 15 drops a day of MMS How many times a day should I take it?

A: Continue taking 15 drops. I think you should take it 2 or 3 times a day for at least a week. Then check to see how your allergies are doing. Then revert to a 6 drops a day maintenance. Oh and remember when you are taking some kind of medicine separate them by three to four hours.

ALS

Has MMS had any success with ALS?

Q: I am wanting to know if you have any knowledge of persons with ALS having any success with MMS treatments. I have ALS and am taking MMS right now (about two weeks) I would like to hear from anyone who has any experience or knowledge of successes with ALS being helped or failure of being helped by MMS treatments

A: I have had a little success, but we have learned a lot of things and I believe that enemas have a better chance in working. I do not know of anyone who used MMS as it is being used on someone who has ALS.

Alzheimer

I would like to know if MMS helps those with Alzheimer's disease?

Q: I would like to know if MMS helps those with Alzheimer's disease?

A: There has been people with Alzheimer who are taking MMS, but we do not know for sure if it helps since they never get back to us. However, MMS has been affecting most diseases positively. We believe that you should go ahead and work with Alzheimer's as MMS doe not cause harm.

Anaerobic

Is there a reaction between DMSO and MMS that you know of?

Q: I received the MMS, and used 2 drops yesterday afternoon. I had used DMSO gel on my knees to help with some stiffness (had knee replacements about 6 months ago) yesterday morning. About 12 hours later I experienced severe itching under the skin around my knees and some slight nausea earlier.

I checked the instructions from GL more closely and noticed that they suggested waiting 72 hours after using DMSO before using MMS, something I had not seen in your instructions. Is there a reaction between DMSO and MMS that you know of? The itching is subsiding this morning, so it's nothing serious but I thought you would want to know about it.

A: Jerome, there is no problem with taking DMSO and MMS. That problem has been settled. No doubt the MMS was attacking some anaerobic growth. It is a good sign.

How does MMS kill the bacteria?

Q: If the MMS kills bacteria, how does it deal with the body's natural bacteria which consists of 80% good and 20% bad? I know you state that it leaves healthy cells and kills the harmful ones, but can it differentiate between bacteria and leave the body's natural bacteria (good and bad) alone? If all the bacteria is destroyed are you promoting a pro-biotic?

A: Good bacteria in the body are known as aerobic bacteria (that means that they use oxygen). Disease causing bacteria are Anaerobic (that means they do not use oxygen). You might suppose then, that there is some sort of difference between them and that is true, there is a difference. Guess what, the unique qualities of the MMS ion (chlorine dioxide) allows it to see the difference between the two different bacteria, and thus it only destroys the anaerobic bacteria (that's the disease causing bacteria). This is also controlled by the white blood cells in the immune system which have the ability to use chlorine dioxide against the diseases.

Animal Treatment

My cat has kidney failure and hyperthyroidism, will MMS help?

Q: I have a 20 yr old cat with a bit of kidney failure and hyperthyroidism. The tapazole that I was giving him for the thyroid has now made him disoriented, head achy and his health seems to be deteriorating fast. I just ordered MMS for him.

1) what is the proper dosage for an 8 lb cat?

2) are there any side effects to watch out for since people sometimes feel nauseous? Do animals respond differently?

3) should I include other supplements?

4) is it ok to give him the thyroid medicines also, although I am stopping them today to see if he improves for now?

5) How do I work around the meat eating issue since he only eats wet food and cannot wait several hours with the allotted dosage times?

A: For animals, take 3 drops of MMS for each 25 pounds of body weight. An 8 pound cat would take 1 drop. Animals respond same as people. I do not normally recommend supplements. That's for doctors or other professionals. Thyroid medicines are ok when separated by several hours from the MMS dose. If you do not have several hours, separate them as far as possible. There really is no meat eating problem. Some people have got that idea erroneously.

What's the recommended dosage for a cat?

Q: What's the recommended dosage for a cat?

A: Here is a way to prepare a dose for a cat. With humans we usually start with one drop and increase to 2 drops and then to 3 drops and so forth. So lets start the same way, but for a cat. Make up a one drop dose (1 drop of MMS, 5 drops of citric acid or lemon, wait 3 minutes, ad 1/2 glass of water). Now a human would drink the whole 1/2 glass, but the cat weighs about 1/00th the amount of a human. So lets take out about 1/2 eye dropper full and give that to the cat. The next time, make up a 2 drop dose and do the same thing. And continue doing it that way until you are making up a 15 drop dose. If the cat gets sick, reduce the dose until the cat is not sick. Keep increasing the doses if you can. Keep up the doses until the cat is well.

How much MMS should I give my cat who is suffering from cancer?

Q: Have a small cat with cancer. Started to give her ½ drop to start. It would be very difficult to put it in 1/3 to 2/3's of liquid. Is that amount necessary? What's the smallest amount I can get away with since I am using an eye dropper to give it to her?

A: Here is a way to prepare a dose for a cat. When treating humans, we usually start with one drop and increase to 2 drops and then to 3 drops and so forth. So lets begin the same way, but for a cat make a one drop dose (1 drop of MMS, 5 drops of citric acid or lemon, wait 3 minutes, ad 1/2 glass of water). Now a human would drink the whole 1/2 glass, but the cat weighs about 1/00th the amount of a human. So lets take out about 1/2 eye dropper full and give that to the cat. The next time, make a 2 drop dose and do the same thing. And continue doing it that way until you are making up a 15 drop dose. If the cat gets sick, reduce the dose until the cat is not sick. Keep increasing the doses if you can. Keep up the doses until the cat is well.

What's the protocol for treating chronic sinus problems and for yeast overgrowth? How can I treat my dog that has Cushing's disease?

Q: Hello. I am interested in taking MMS for chronic sinus problems and for yeast overgrowth. I would also like to give it to my dog that has Cushing's disease. I am going to order MMS, but would like to know a recommended dosage for my 8 lb. Maltese.

A: Do the standard protocol. For animals, use 3 drops for every 25 pounds of body weight.

How long should we stay on a 15 drops a day dose before we go to maintenance?

Q: I am on 15 drops a day and feel stronger and happier every day. My 75 lb golden retriever is on 9 drops a day. How long should we stay on this amount before we go to maintenance? With my dog I put 9 drops with 45 drops of lime juice to activate the MMS then after 3 minutes I mix the solution with organic chicken broth and dog food is that ok?

A: For you and your dog stay at that dose for 1 week. After that, do the maintenance dose. This is from 4 to 6 drops a day for older people and 4 to 6 drops twice a week for younger people. I would prefer if she took it with only water, but if you just need the soup, you can add 2 teaspoons of citric acid solution or lemon juice to the soup to make it acid. The 45 drops of acid that you used for the MMS is not enough for the soup too, so use the extra acid. The dog will be able to drink it OK.

How can I treat my cocker spaniel puppy for cancer?

Q: I have a cocker spaniel puppy 24 Lbs recently diagnosed with Mast Cell Tumors level 2 cancer. Do you think it would also be healthy and beneficial for my best friend? I can not stand the thought of losing her, she is only 20 months old. If you think it would be safe how much should I give her? The standard 2 drops to start?

A: Here is a way to prepare a dose for a pet. With humans we usually start with one drop and increase to 2 drops and then to 3 drops and so forth. So lets start the same way, but for a cat. Make up a one drop dose (1 drop of MMS, 5 drops of citric acid or lemon, wait 3 minutes, ad 1/2 glass of water). Now a human would drink the whole 1/2 glass, but the pet weighs less than a human. So lets take out about the percentage that the animal weights in relation to the human. If the pet weighs 1/10th as much as the human, take out 1/10th the amount of liquid and give it to the pet. The next time, make up a 2 drop dose and do the same thing. And continue doing it that way until you are making up a 15 drop dose. If the pet gets sick, reduce the dose until the pet is not sick. Keep increasing the doses if you can. Keep up the doses until the pet is well.

What is the protocol for livestock?

Q: What is the protocol for livestock?

A: For animals the dose is 3 drops for every 25 pounds.

Have you any information about using MMS for worms in cats and dogs?

Q: Have you any information about using MMS for worms in cats and dogs? What dosage would be used for drops/Kg weight? Would it be effective?

A: For pets use 3 drops for every 25 pounds of body weight. We have had many good reports.

How much water or juice should I add to the activated MMS to treat a cat with kidney failure?

Q: I am not clear about whether it matters how much water or juice you add to the activated MMS.

I want to treat a cat with kidney failure and can get a 1/2 a syringe of activated MMS in a 1/2 teaspoon of water into her is this adequate or is there a danger in taking too little liquid with the MMS?

Please explain the logic. Could I kill my cat if the toxin load discharges, since the kidneys have to process it?

A: Here is a way to prepare a dose for a cat. With humans we usually start with one drop and increase to two drops and then to three drops and so forth. So, lets start the same way, but for a cat. First, make a one drop dose (1 drop of MMS, 5 drops of citric acid or lemon, wait 3 minutes, add 1/2 glass of water). Now a human would drink the whole 1/2 glass, but the cat weighs about 1/00th the amount of a human. So lets take out about 1/2 eye dropper full and give that to the cat. Next time, make a two drop dose and do the same thing. Continue doing it that way until you are making a 15 drop dose. If the cat gets sick, reduce the dose until the cat is not sick. Keep increasing the doses if you can. Keep up the doses until the cat is well.

How many drops can I give my dog? Is it OK to feel nauseous and get cold chills after taking 6 drops of MMS?

Q: How many drops can I give my dog? He weighs 80 lbs. Also I am taking 6 drops a day and I am currently on my 9th day and I have been feeling slightly dizzy nauseous and get cold chills can I stay at 6 drops per day?

A: For pets the correct dose is 3 drops per every 25 pounds.

Add the citric acid, let it sit for three minutes then add 1/2 glass of water and give it to the dog. Yes, it is ok to stay at 6 drops. That is the maintenance dose. If you feel a little nausea just lower the dose a little bit so that you are not feeling nauseous. Keep attempting to increase the dose but only when you think the nausea is gone. Keep attempting to increase the dose in this way until you have reached 15 drops at least twice a day.

Is it better to give a pet the MMS on an empty or full stomach?

Q: I am treating a dog diagnosed with lymphoma. I am doing an aggressive treatment 3 drops per 25 lbs. I wanted to ask you if its better to give the treatment before or after eating?

A: MMS is more effective on an empty stomach, however, because of this effectiveness, your pet is very likely to experience nausea. By eating prior to taking MMS there will be less nausea. You are doing well. If the dog does not get nauseous with 3 drops go to 4 or more and maintain the dosage. As for cancer, always go with as much MMS as possible.

I have a small cat with cancer. How much MMS can I give her?

Q: I have a small cat with cancer. How much MMS can I give her?

A: Here is a way to prepare a dose for a pet. With humans we usually start with one drop and increase to 2 drops and then to

3 drops and so forth. So lets start the same way, but in this case it will be for a cat. Make a one drop dose (1 drop of MMS, 5 drops of citric acid or lemon, wait 3 minutes, ad 1/2 glass of water). Now a human would drink the whole 1/2 glass, but the pet weighs less than a human. So lets take out about the percentage that the animal weights in relation to the human. If the pet weighs 1/10th as much as the human, take out 1/10th the amount of liquid and give it to the pet. The next time, make up a 2 drop dose and do the same thing. And continue doing it that way until you are making up a 15 drop dose. If the pet gets sick, reduce the dose until the pet is not sick. Keep increasing the doses if you can. Keep up the doses until the pet is well.

Will MMS help my two-month old puppy to fight megaesophagus that might lead to pneumonia?

Q: We have been given a 2 month old puppy with what they call megaesophagus that apparently can lead to pneumonia. I want to know if you think MMS would help the mega-e as well as the pneumonia in the event that he gets that. How would I go about giving the puppy a maintenance dose in the meantime. Could I put it in goat's milk. He loves that but does not drink water much.

A: MMS will overcome that problem. Here is a way to prepare a dose for a pet. With humans we usually start with one drop and increase to 2 drops and then to 3 drops and so forth. So lets start the same way. For a cat, make up a one drop dose (1 drop of MMS, 5 drops of citric acid or lemon, wait 3 minutes, ad 1/2 glass of water). Now a human would drink the whole 1/2 glass, but the pet weighs less than a human; so lets take out about the percentage that the animal weights in relation to the human. If the pet weighs 1/10th as much as the human, take out 1/10th the amount of liquid and give it to the pet. Use an eye dropper. The next time, make a 2 drop dose and do the same thing. Continue doing it that way until you are taking a 15 drop dose. If the pet gets sick, reduce the dose until the pet is not sick. Keep increasing the doses if you can. Keep up the doses until the pet is well.

How can I get Chlorine Dioxide to treat my dog?

Q: There is "something" inside my dog, I had her treated for tape worm. Do you think I could use it on her and get rid of the beast in her once and for all? Also, I am a bit confused... would I treat her with drops of SODIUM CHLORITE or mix per instructions to get CHLORINE DIOXIDE and treat her with that? Please advise and thanks for any info you can give me.

A: Chlorine dioxide is generated from sodium chlorite with the addition of a food acid. Follow the same procedure as the standard protocol as described in my web site and remember that for animals, the dose is 3 drops for each 25 pounds of body weight. That's 1 drop for each 8 pounds of body weight. But do not start out with that much. Follow the procedure.

What is the recommended dose for animals?

Q: Can you tell me what dose would be good for an animal (cat) this size and how to give it to her?

A: Dear Gary, For animals, give them 3 drops of MMS for

every 25 pounds, for each drop of MMS, put 5 drops of citric acid, wait 3 minutes then add half glass of water. It's ok if they do not drink it all, for it can probably last from 20 to 24 hours; so it is ok for them to drink it through out the day. If they will not drink it, use a turkey baster or eye dropper for a small animal.

Is it OK to mix a dosage of MMS for my cattle and pour it over two handfuls of grain so that he eats it immediately?

Q: I have a head of cattle that has a bad infection on the back of it's rear leg. It has swollen up pretty bad. His weight is about 1700-2000 lbs. I have been giving him 150 drops twice a day. The question is… Is it OK to mix up the MMS, wait the 3 minutes and then pour it over two handfuls of grain (feed) so that he eats it immediately? He then generally takes a nice big drink of water (about 5 gallons). Let me know what you think about this "pouring the MMS over a couple of hand fulls of grain".

A: Dear Martin, I think it is best for you to give it to your cattle in the water. Remember, for animals give 3 drops of MMS for every 25 pounds of body weight. When mixing MMS, let say your cattle weights 1700 pounds, that would be 204 MMS drops with 1020 drops of citric acid, wait 3 minutes and pour that to the animal's water. The cattle can drink it throughout the day. What you can also do is spray some in its infected area. To do this, take a 2 ounce bottle, add 20 drops of MMS, mix it with 100 drops of citric acid, wait 3 minutes and pour it to the 2 ounce bottle; add some water to that solution then spray the affected area.

Does having breakfast affect my MMS treatment? Can I also use MMS on my puppy?

Q: Could you please tell me if I can take MMS in the morning and still have breakfast which includes milk and cereal? I also have a Newfoundland 11 month old puppy who has severe allergies and I believe she has a yeast infection, Can I give it to her and how much should I start her on, many, many thanks. Shirley.

A: Dear Sophie, yes, you can take MMS after eating. Just wait a couple of minutes. I always suggest people to wait 1 or 2 hours, but that is only because MMS works better on an empty stomach. You can also give some to your puppy. Three drops of MMS for every 25 pounds of body weight, remember that for each drop of MMS you should add 5 drops of citric acid, lime or lemon juice, wait 3 minutes and then add water to it.

For how long should I continue with a dosage of MMS If I already feel better?

Q: How long is it ok for me to do 8 drops daily and my 80 pound dog 5 drops daily? We all feel better on these dosages

A: You can take it as long as you are feeling ok, but you are going to eventually have to take the maintenance dose, which is 4 or 6 drops a day for older people (+50) and 4 to 6 drops twice a week for younger people.

How much MMS is required for a small cat with cancer?

Q: I have a small cat with cancer. How much MMS can I give her?

A: Here is a way to prepare a dose for a pet. With humans we usually start with one drop and increase to 2 drops and then to 3 drops and so forth. So lets start the same way, but for a cat. Make up a one drop dose (1 drop of MMS, 5 drops of citric acid or lemon, wait 3 minutes, ad 1/2 glass of water). Now a human would drink the whole 1/2 glass, but the pet weighs less than a human. So lets take out about the percentage that the animal weights in relation to the human. If the pet weighs 1/10th as much as the human, take out 1/10th the amount of liquid and give it to the pet. The next time, make up a 2 drop dose and do the same thing. And continue doing it that way until you are making up a 15 drop dose. If the pet gets sick, reduce the dose until the pet is not sick. Keep increasing the doses if you can. Keep up the doses until the pet is well.

Ankylosing Spondolitis

Will MMS work on Hep C, Thrombocytopenia, Leukytosis, Crohn's Disease, Ankylosing Spondolitis, Osteopenia, Chronic severe Insomnia and Inflammatory, Rheumatoid, Degenerative and Osteoarthritis?

Q: I have Hep C, Thrombocytopenia, Leukytosis, Crohn's Disease, Ankylosing Spondolitis, Osteopenia, Chronic severe Insomnia and Inflammatory, Rheumatoid, Degenerative and Osteoarthritis. Will I be able to use this product safely?

A: Yes you will be able to use MMS safely if you follow the protocol starting off with 1/2 drop of MMS. Go to one of my sites listed below and follow the standard protocol, but be very slow to go to each new increase of MMS. Remember, when you feel sick, just lower the dose a few drops. MMS will help you with many of your diseases.

Antibiotics

Can MMS help me with gut parasites?

Q: I have been suffering for years with gut parasites, giardia was found in my stool some years ago. Antibiotics have proved ineffective but, I have reduced the infection down greatly with herbal methods. The reason I am writing to you is because I am undecided as to the dose I should start off with. In your book you state that one should always start with one drop and build up except in the case of a parasitic problem in which case start at 15 drops. Also, what is the procedure, if nausea comes on too strong or vomiting takes place, as to the second dose of the day? Do I reduce back to one drop and work back up, or just say halve the dose? Finally, because gut parasites are not in the blood, can the immune system aided by the MMS still seek them out?

A: Always start off with 1 drop of MMS 2 or 3 times a day. Increase 1 drop per day until you get to 15 drops 2 or 3 times a day. When you start feeling sick (nausea, vomiting, headache or diarrhea), just lower the dose to the point where you are not feeling bad, once you overcome those symptoms start increasing the dose. What MMS finds it will kill it.

Do I need to brush with baking soda after using MMS? Will there be a conflict if a person is also taking cumadin, lipitor or other RX including like leavaquin or cipro

antibiotics?

Q: Someone said we need to brush with baking soda after using MMS? Will there be a conflict if a person is also taking cumadin, lipitor or other RX including like leavaquin or cipro antibiotics?

A: You do not have to use baking soda after brushing with MMS. You use MMS as a normal tooth paste and you can use it as a mouth wash as well. If the person is taking some kind of drug or medicine, just wait from 2 to 3 hours apart. MMS does not conflict with Medicines.

Is it a good idea to use MMS while taking antibiotics?

Q: Is it a good idea to use MMS while taking antibiotics?

A: You can take MMS and other medications 4 hours apart.

What is the most effective way to take MMS to fight Chronic fatigue & immune dysfunction syndrome?

Q: I started MMS treatment two nights ago. I put 2 drops in a cup, mixed 1/2 teaspoon of lime juice. Waited for 3 minutes. Added 1/3 cup of water. I want to make sure I am doing this right. I have very severe CFIDS (chronic fatigue and immune dysfunction syndrome), and I am totally bedridden much of the time. Also several docs feel I have late stage Lyme disease on top of it as well as metals. Can this help me? I did not tolerate 3 months of antibiotics at all. It seems like MMS also kills many bacteria. What about viruses and bacteria that hide out in cells and replicate in ways that the immune system does not find them? Can this help?

A: For every drop of MMS you need to add 5 drops of citric acid, lime or lemon juice. Wait 3 minutes and add half a glass of water or juice. So far the most effective way is to take 3 or 4 drops 3 or 4 times a day. A lot of people who have Lyme disease have taken MMS and it seems to help quite a bit, but no one has said that there are completely cured. I only have 2 people that have said they are cured. I personally had people tested for heavy metals before and after taking MMS, and the heavy metals were reduced significantly or totally gone after 2 weeks.

Antioxidants and Proteins

How far apart should we take MMS from antioxidants?

Q: I have been sent this question what do you say? I have a question regarding antioxidants. I have read that all antioxidants negate the effects of MMS, not just Vitamin C. If I take MMS 3x/day and should take no antioxidants 3 hours before and 3 hours after the MMS dosage, that pretty well leaves out any window for anything but the MMS. Would you please comment on this? Should antioxidants be put aside or still used? If so, when?

A: I do not know how much antioxidants affect MMS, but I would wait at least 2 hour before and after taking antioxidants to take MMS. That's a 4 hour window in a day. That leaves 20 hours out of 24 for other things. If you have a specific antioxidant in mind, if you will send me several pills I will test them to see if it affects the MMS.

How long apart should we take MMS from animal proteins and antioxidants?

Q: One of our Study members who are taking MMS and sulfur is also taking bio identical hormones for her thyroid and antioxidants. Her practitioner has told her to take the MMS apart from animal proteins and antioxidants. Can you add to this discussion? We have suggested that she take the sulfur first being that we have demonstrated that the sulfur transports across the stomach blood barrier into the lymph within 30 minutes.

A: It is my practice to suggest the MMS be separated in time by at least one hour when taking other things.

Arthritis

Arthritis and MMS

Q: I was extremely disappointed with the description you give to Arthritis. In four years that I studied nutrition never came across with your description. Basically, the term 'arthritis' describes the inflammation of a joint, or joints. The chief forms are osteoarthritis and rheumatoid arthritis, and the underlying cause of both is too much uric acid in the body.

A: Just to give a little more information, when the muscles in the various parts of the body begin acting up and the wrong muscles try to move the body part, it creates stress that causes inflammation. That, in turn causes various kinds of bacteria or viruses to catch hold and begin growing in that area. The fact that literally thousands of people have been cured by simply doing the unusual exercises given in the book, does not mean that the same condition cannot be cured with nutrition. In dealing with the thousands of people that have used MMS over the past 10 years, I have come to realize that a lot of nutrition is based not on nutrition for the body, but rather in not feeding the parasite, bacteria, viral, mold, yeast, load that the body has. When that load has been killed by MMS, the body begins to repair all the damage done. It can then utilize many kinds of nutrients that it could not use before. It repairs quickly. Please do not believe anything I say. Just try it.

Could you please tell me if MMS will do any harm to the red blood cells since I have Beta Thalassemia Minor? Would it help my being anemic?

Q: I have a inherited Blood Disease "Beta Thalassemia Minor" in which my red blood cells are smaller and odd shaped from normal red blood cells. This causes me to be Anemic and I will always be anemic. Could you please tell me if MMS will do any harm to the red blood cells? I would really like to try MMS because of back problems, and arthritis. And would it help my being anemic?

A: MMS does not harm red blood cells. It will probably help the disease as well as your arthritis.

Will MMS help with arthritis, inflammation in my foot and some pain in my hand that might be carpal tunnel syndrome?

Q: My daughter had me order some MMS. I have had horrible pain in my left hand, elbow and arm it could be carpal tunnel syndrome, but I have had that before and this just feels different. Will MMS help? I also found out that I have arthritis and inflammation in my foot can MMS help this? Can I use 100% cherry juice?

A: Yes. It will help you there have been good results for inflammation and arthritis. Just make sure the juice does not contain Vitamin C (ascorbic acid) then it is ok to use.

Can MMS help me with arthritis and inflammation in my foot?

Q: I have arthritis and inflammation in my foot can MMS help this? Can I use 100% cherry juice?

A: Yes it will help you there have been good results for inflammation and arthritis. Just make sure the juice does not contain Vitamin C (ascorbic acid), and is it ok to use.

Will MMS assist with diabetes, arthritis, stroke victims and constipation?

Q: Will MMS assist with diabetes, arthritis, stroke victims and constipation?

A: Yes it will help all of those conditions.

Can I take MMS while on Methotrexate, Celebrex and armor thyroid?

Q: I have Rheumatoid Arthritis and take Methotrexate, Celebrex and armor thyroid. Wondering if I can take with the medicines I am on?

A: Yes, you can keep taking your medications, just wait 3 to 4 hours after taking MMS.

Do you have any experience with treating the arthritis with MMS?

Q: I have suffered with rheumatoid arthritis and fibromyalgia for the past 20 years, I am 49 now. Do you have any experience with treating the arthritis with MMS?

A: A number of people have phoned or emailed me saying that they had gotten relief from arthritis and fibromyalgia. However, with figromyalgia it is important to eat breakfast within half an hour after waking and to continue to eat many small meals during the day.

Does MMS do any harm to red blood cells?

Q: I have an inherited Blood Disease "Beta Thalassemia Minor" in which my red blood cells are smaller and odd shaped from normal red blood cells. This causes me to be Anemic and I will always be anemic. Could you please tell me if MMS will do any harm to the red blood cells? I would really like to try MMS because of back problems, and arthritis.

A: MMS does not harm red blood cells. It will probably help the disease as well as your back problems and arthritis.

Could you help me with suggestions concerning dosages and usage of the MMS and water combo package for

92

maximum benefit?

Q: I would be grateful for your suggestions concerning dosages/usage of the MMS and the water combo package with the Prill beads & balls for maximum benefit:

Person #1 is recovering from breast cancer, is a smoker, and has undergone chemo: Person #2 is paraplegic with chronic bladder/kidney infections [also ordered colloidal silver for him], asthma and allergies, anxiety attacks and chronic depression, suspected add or onset of bipolar disorder: Person #3 is type 2 diabetic, high blood pressure, high cholesterol, degenerative arthritic condition, chronic obesity.

A: All these people you mention should follow the standard protocol for MMS. Start with two drops MMS, add ten drops of lemon or lime or citric acid solution as described in my book, mix, allow to set three minutes, add 1/2 glass or water and drink. Go the three drops, then to four, and then to 5, each time always using the correct amount of lemon or lime or citric. If nausea occurs, take a drop or two less next time. Then keep increasing the drops until you have reached 15 drops a day for 5 or 6 days then increase to three 15 drop doses a day until the problem is gone. Do not remain at three 15 drop doses a day for longer than 2 months. Reduce the amount as soon as possible. Then decrease to 4 to 6 drops a day for maintenance.

Will MMS work on Hep C, Thrombocytopenia, Leukytosis, Crohn's Disease, Ankylosing Spondolitis, Osteopenia, Chronic severe Insomnia and Inflammatory,

Rheumatoid, Degenerative and Osteoarthritis?

Q: I have Hep C, Thrombocytopenia, Leukytosis, Crohn's Disease, Ankylosing Spondolitis, Osteopenia, Chronic severe Insomnia and Inflammatory, Rheumatoid, Degenerative and Osteoarthritis. Will I be able to use this product safely?

A: Yes you will be able to use MMS safely if you follow the protocol starting off with 1/2 drop of MMS. Go to one of my sites listed below and follow the standard protocol, but be very slow to go to each new increase of MMS. Remember, when you feel sick, just lower the dose a few drops. MMS will help you with many of your diseases.

Can MMS harm Red Blood Cells in an Anemic patient?

Q: I would really like to try MMS because of back problems and arthritis.

However I have an inherited Blood Disease "Beta Thalassemia Minor" in which my red blood cells are smaller and odd shaped from normal red blood cells. This causes me to be Anemic and I will always be anemic. Could you please tell me if MMS will do any harm to the red blood cells?

A: MMS does not harm red blood cells. Most likely, it will help the disease as well as your back problems and arthritis.

Back Problems

Will MMS have a bad reaction if I am currently taking medication?

Q: 3 years ago I fell and injured by spinal cord at T-12. I take baclofen (spasms) and neurontin (nerve pain) at 6am, 2pm and again at 10pm. I also take vicodin throughout the day for breakthrough pain. If I take MMS at 10 am, what problem do you think will I have by taking vicodin before 2?

A: MMS does not have bad reactions to medications. It is ok if you leave 2, 3 or 4 hours apart, just try to pattern your doses.

Does MMS do any harm to red blood cells?

Q: I have an inherited Blood Disease "Beta Thalassemia Minor" in which my red blood cells are smaller and odd shaped from normal red blood cells. This causes me to be Anemic and I will always be anemic. Could you please tell me if MMS will do any harm to the red blood cells? I would really like to try MMS because of back problems, and arthritis.

A: MMS does not harm red blood cells. It will probably help the disease as well as your back problems and arthritis.

Can MMS harm Red Blood Cells in an Anemic patient?

Q: I would really like to try MMS because of back problems and arthritis.

However I have an inherited Blood Disease "Beta Thalassemia Minor" in which my red blood cells are smaller and odd shaped from normal red blood cells. This causes me to be Anemic and I will always be anemic. Could you please tell me if MMS will do any harm to the red blood cells?

A: MMS does not harm red blood cells. Most likely, it will help the disease as well as your back problems and arthritis.

Bacteria

Does MMS help Heart Attacks?

Q: Does MMS help Heart Attacks?

A: A number of people have reported that their heart condition was improved since beginning to take MMS. One man who was having small heart attacks every day was no more having heart attacks after taking the MMS for three days. Several persons who began having heart palpitations after taking MMS reported later that they felt that their heart was in better condition. The palpitations could be caused by killing bacteria growth on the heart valve.

I would like to know what MMS does to good bacteria in the blood. Does MMS also kill them?

Q: I would like to know what MMS does to good bacteria in the blood. Does MMS also kill them?

A: MMS does not touch good bacteria nor does it kill good cells.

If I got sick by taking 5 drops of MMS should I increase this dose or lower it?

Q: I have suffered with chronic fungal infections and bacterial infections and have mercury poising for ten years. I have tried MMS but it made me sick at 2 drops should I take more or less?

A: Stay at 2 drops for a week, then start increasing the drops 1 a day so you can pass the 2 drops you have to go all the way up to 15 drops, but on your way to the 15 drops if you get sick again lower the dosage, remember that when you get nauseous or diarrhea is a good indicator which means you are eliminating some bad stuff from you system. Also it's OK to take MMS if you have mercury, do not worry about that it will get rid of it. But remember your goal is to go up to 15 drops 2 or 3 times a day for a week. Then after a week go to the maintenance dose.

What is the most effective way to take MMS to fight Chronic fatigue & immune dysfunction syndrome?

Q: I started MMS treatment two nights ago. I put 2 drops in a cup, mixed 1/2 teaspoon of lime juice. Waited for 3 minutes. Added 1/3 cup of water. I want to make sure I am doing this right. I have very severe CFIDS (chronic fatigue and immune dysfunction syndrome), and I am totally bedridden much of the time. Also several docs feel I have late stage Lyme disease on top of it as well as metals. Can this help me? I did not tolerate 3 months of antibiotics at all. It seems like MMS also kills many bacteria. What about viruses and bacteria that hide out in cells and replicate in ways that the immune system does not find them? Can this help?

A: For every drop of MMS you need to add 5 drops of citric acid, lime or lemon juice. Wait 3 minutes and add half a glass of water or juice. So far the most effective way is to take 3 or 4 drops 3 or 4 times a day. A lot of people who have Lyme disease have taken MMS and it seems to help quite a bit, but no one has said that there are completely cured. I only have 2 people that have said they are cured. I personally had people tested for heavy metals before and after taking MMS, and the heavy metals were reduced significantly or totally gone after 2 weeks.

How does MMS kill the bacteria?

Q: If the MMS kills bacteria, how does it deal with the body's natural bacteria which consists of 80% good and 20% bad? I know you state that it leaves healthy cells and kills the harmful ones, but can it differentiate between bacteria and leave the body's natural bacteria (good and bad) alone? If all the bacteria is destroyed are you promoting a pro-biotic?

A: Good bacteria in the body are known as aerobic bacteria (that means that they use oxygen). Disease causing bacteria are Anaerobic (that means they do not use oxygen). You might suppose then, that there is some sort of difference between them and that is true, there is a difference. Guess what, the unique qualities of the MMS ion (chlorine dioxide) allows it to see the difference between the two different bacteria, and thus it only destroys the anaerobic bacteria (that's the disease causing bacteria). This is also controlled by the white blood cells in the immune system which have the ability to use chlorine dioxide against the diseases.

Bartonella

Would MMS help the lyme if bartonella is also there?

Q: I am new to the lyme world. I was diagnosed with CFS and sick for 24 years. Now my 24 year old daughter is sick with lyme and bartonella or mycoplasma. (what I now know, I probably have lyme too.) Would MMS help the lyme if bartonella is also there?

And, right now she chose to start cumanda and samento before she goes on an antibiotic, would MMS fit into this regime?

One last question, if you would not mind, how does MMS differ from the Salt/C protocol?

My daughter is on DHEA and testosterone cream, midodrine due to low blood pressure (I am not sure if it is working) and salt tablets. She just started cumanda and samento because she is doing school 5 days a week and is afraid of herx from antibiotics since she is getting married in August and has Bar exam in July.

A: MMS is chlorine dioxide, an oxidizer that kills pathogens, but does not touch the rest of the body. It is totally different from the salt and vitamin C action. At this point I do not know anything that is guaranteed in handling lyme. MMS has proved effective depending upon the protocol and the person. It occurs to me that salt seems to drive the lyme out into the open, and the salt might work well with MMS. So the state of the lyme protocol is still being tested by many different people. But in my opinion, the best weapon so far is MMS and chemistry does not have a better weapon even in theory.

What do you recommend for a person who has been

experiencing depression, irritability, brain fog and fatigue due to Lyme disease?

Q: I have Lyme disease and many of its co-infections; bartonella, babesia and ehrlichia, to name the big ones. I have been taking MMS for two weeks, but have only managed to get up to five drops, twice a day, because I am experiencing increased depression, irritability, brain fog and fatigue. (No nausea whatsoever though). I am tempted to ramp up faster per your instructions, but I fear the depression could get out of control. I am surprised that after two weeks, I only feel worse instead of better. My questions are: Has the same thing happened to other Lyme sufferers? What would you recommend as far as dosing? Do you think I could have detoxification problems and this is why I am not improving, or is the MMS just killing a lot of bugs? Also, do you know if MMS can get Lyme in cystic form?

A: Most people who have Lyme disease have similar reactions, take less MMS keep the dose down to where you can tolerate it, the MMS Will handle most of the side disease and we are still working on a Lyme protocol other than what I am suggesting here, we are working and in my opinion you would have to go intervenes treatment before Lyme will be completely cured.

Blood

Does MMS reduce serum iron in the blood?

Q: My problem is iron overload and I have to give blood every 60 days. I have been taking MMS since Dec. 26, 2007. Seeing that iron is a mineral, does MMS reduce serum iron in the blood?

A: MMS reduces in water supply's but I really do not know if it reduces it in the blood, I have to look into that. Thank you for pointing it out.

Can an 87 year old man with a pacemaker and on blood thinners take MMS?

Q: Is it possible for an 87 year old man with a pacemaker and on blood thinners to take MMS?

A: Yes, it is possible, just start out very slowly. I start with 1/2 drop the first day. Look for negative effects, and then go to 1 drop. Negative effects do not mean that there is a problem because killing pathogens creates poisons in the system. But if you notice a problem with the pacemaker do not increase, but do not stop. The MMS does not affect metals and other items. It only kills the pathogens. Just go slow.

I have some questions, can you answer them please?

Q: 1. Are there particle clumping problems over time? 2. I have DMSO to use as a vehicle through the skin; are there other means of carrying the Ag into nerve tissues? 3. What amounts s/be used for various treatments? Questions 1 and 3 will determine purchase amounts.

A: There are no particle clumping problems. There is niacin to help carry MMS into the body. Take enough to turn your skin red. That is caused by the blood vessels enlarging.

Does MMS Clear clogging from the arteries of the body?

Q: Does MMS Clear clogging from the arteries of the body?

A: One lady called to say that she was in very bad shape. Her doctor had told her that her arteries more than 80% clogged. He could not say how much more because one cannot measure more than 80% accurately.

She worked up to 15 drops three times a day and then did that for 30 days. When she was retested her reading was less than 50% clogged. Several other people have mentioned that their clogged readings were reduced. That's what people have called or emailed to say. I believe it.

How do we go about intravenous MMS for HIV patients?

Q: You mentioned giving intravenous MMS to HIV patients. How do we go about it? How many drops (15?) mixed with sterile water?(No citric acid of course). To what proportions? How frequently? And for children? Do the orally doses work well with HIV patients?

A: Do not use sterile water. Us IV solution either saline or glucose or other sugar solutions sold for that purpose. Normally the glucose works best as the saline sometimes causes a drop in blood pressure. If you use a 500 ML bottle start with one drop. Wait and hour after adding the MMS to allow for activation. Use one drop the first day, two drops the second day. Then increase to 6 or 8 the third day. Then increase by 4 to 8 drops a day until you are doing 22 drops in

500 ML of solution in a 2 to 4 hour drip. Normally you would do it until the person is well. Sometimes it works good with HIV patients orally and sometimes you need to do intravenous.

Is it possible to get infection at 15 drops of MMS treatment?

Q: I have been taking the drops for the last couple of months, I have a lot of health issues, diabetes, blood pressure and kidneys and prostate, the worse is exhaustion most of the time. I got to 15 drops and 10 drops within 2 to 4 hrs, I had to cut down, it was very hard getting out of bed in the morning. I am taking 15 drops for couple of weeks. The most interesting, had two prostate infections while at 15 drops, I had to resort to the Beck devise to clear the infection, is it possible to get infection at 15 drops? What do you think of all this?

A: First of all you must increase the drops 1 by 1 each day not all at once, when you start feeling bad you have to cut down the drops and when you are feeling better you must increase the drops. When you get up to 15 drops only take it for 1 week and stay at 6 drops once a day.

Can MMS cause lower blood pressure?

Q: Can MMS cause lower blood pressure? My mom has taken MMS for about 5 days. She started with 1 drop, 2x a day. She is now on 5 drops 2x a day. Her blood pressure dropped from 80/50 five days ago to 58/50 today. I am concerned. Should she stop taking MMS or is there something she can do to raise the pressure while on MMS?

A: Drink a glass of apple or pine apple or cranberry juice or grape juice, drink a full glass of juice before and after taking MMS within 10 minutes before and after, and that should keep her blood pressure level up, if it do not she should increase her drops until her blood pressure do not go down.

Could you please tell me if MMS will do any harm to the red blood cells since I have Beta Thalassemia Minor? Would it help my being anemic?

Q: I have a inherited Blood Disease "Beta Thalassemia Minor" in which my red blood cells are smaller and odd shaped from normal red blood cells. This causes me to be Anemic and I will always be anemic. Could you please tell me if MMS will do any harm to the red blood cells? I would really like to try MMS because of back problems, and arthritis. And would it help my being anemic?

A: MMS does not harm red blood cells. It will probably help the disease as well as your arthritis.

Should I continue increasing my MMS dosage if I am starting to have stomach cramping while treating parasites?

Q: How do I know how long to take it after I reach 15 drops once a day? I have had parasites due to a bird mite infestation and want to strengthen my immune system. I also have high cholesterol so I want to take it for that. I am up to 9 drops and am experiencing diarrhea and stomach cramping. I know it says this is a normal reaction, but should I continue increasing the dosage?

A: Stay 1 week at 15 drops (if you are well you can take it 2 or 3 times day) after that week stay at the maintenance dose which is 4 or 6 drops a day for older people and 4 to 6 drops twice a week for younger people. When you experience diarrhea, nausea, or vomiting just lower the dose to 1 or 2 drops when this stops starts increasing the dose again until you get pass that sickness.

If my white cells are elevated and my red blood cells too low was it caused by using MMS?

Q: My doc called me because for some strange reason, my white cells were elevated, the red blood cells were too low and it showed that I am anemic. I have not had these problems before and I am wondering if somehow it was connected to the MMS? Any experience with this?

A: No one has ever mentioned this so far over 10 years and thousands of emails. I doubt it. You could stop the MMS and take high levels of B12 for a while, maybe 2 weeks, and see what your blood looks like. Hopefully the anemic reading will be OK or better. Or you could just continue with the MMS and see if the anemic condition improves. Or you could stop the MMS for a week or so and then check the condition to see if the MMS was depressing the reading for some reason.

What do you recommend for a person who has been experiencing depression, irritability, brain fog and fatigue due to Lyme disease?

Q: I have Lyme disease and many of its co-infections; bartonella, babesia and ehrlichia, to name the big ones. I have been taking MMS for two weeks, but have only managed to get up to five drops, twice a day, because I am experiencing increased depression, irritability, brain fog and fatigue. (No nausea whatsoever though). I am tempted to ramp up faster per your instructions, but I fear the depression could get out of control. I am surprised that after two weeks, I only feel worse instead of better. My questions are: Has the same thing happened to other Lyme sufferers? What would you recommend as far as dosing? Do you think I could have detoxification problems and this is why I am not improving, or is the MMS just killing a lot of bugs? Also, do you know if MMS can get Lyme in cystic form?

A: Most people who have Lyme disease have similar reactions, take less MMS keep the dose down to where you can tolerate it, the MMS Will handle most of the side disease and we are still working on a Lyme protocol other than what I am suggesting here, we are working and in my opinion you would have to go intervenes treatment before Lyme will be completely cured.

How many drops should I really need to take to get rid of Lyme disease coupled with Babesia?

Q: I have Lyme disease coupled with Babesia and who knows what other co-infections are probably raging in me. Can this really cure me? How many drops should I really need to take?

A: A lot of people that have contracted Lyme disease are taking MMS and it seems to help quite a bit but no one has said that there completely cured. I only have 2 people that have said they are cured. You must start out at 1 drop per day, you can take it 2 or 3 times a day, increase the drops 1 a day when you start getting nausea or get diarrhea lower the dosage, then when you get well keep increasing the drops until you get to 15 drops, There is a lot of people that take more than 15 drops but that depends on them. Everyone reacts differently.

Is it advisable to take MMS while under high blood pressure medication (TOPROL)?

Q: Is it advisable to take MMS while under high blood pressure medication (TOPROL)?

A: Take MMS and medication 4 hours apart; remember that MMS is only in your body for less than an hour.

Can you positively tell me that MMS will not affect my blood pressure condition?

Q: Can you positively tell me that MMS will not affect my blood pressure condition?

A: No it will not affect you.

Can MMS cause lower blood pressure?

Q: My mom has taken MMS for about 5 days. She started with 1 drop, 2x a day. She is now on 5 drops 2x a day. Her blood pressure dropped from 80/50 five days ago to 58/50 today. I am concerned. Should she stop taking MMS or is there something she can do to raise the pressure while on MMS?

A: Drink a glass of apple or pine apple or cranberry juice or grape juice, drink a full glass of juice before and after taking MMS within 10 minutes before and after, and that should keep her blood pressure level up, if it does not she should increase her drops until her blood pressure goes down.

Is it normal that MMS seems to lower my blood pressure and body energy?

Q: I started taking MMS a few days ago and was able to work up to 3 drops once per day. I am in good health and have been taking vitamin supplements for years. I would like to know if MMS sometimes causes adverse reactions not pertaining to detoxification symptoms such as nausea or diarrhea. I have not experienced any nausea or diarrhea but I noticed that the MMS tends to lower my blood pressure while increasing my heart rate. I was taking 3 drops only once per day in the afternoon and when it was time for bed my heart rate or pulse was still around 100 which prevented me from sleeping. I would wake up feeling groggy with no energy.

A: If you blood pressure goes low drink a glass of homemade fruit juice for the grogginess and the other indication is that something is being killed, destroyed in your body, you will not receive indications otherwise MMS is not a nutrient it does not supply any nutrients to your body. The other nutrients that you are taking for your immune system are very good MMS only supplies a killer to your immune system making it many times mores effectiveness so try right after you take MMS eat a couple of apples that should over come your grogginess but do not quit taking MMS.

Is it the fact that MMS eventually turns to table salt

harmful for patients with high blood pressure or heart problems?

Q: After a period of 12 hours, the MMS turns to table salt. Is not this harmful for high blood pressure or heart problems?

A: MMS turns to approx. 10 ml of table salt that is about 1/2 the size of a pin head you could probably not taste it in a half glass of water, and besides all that the idea that salt causes high blood pressure is just a fable of modern medicine.

Does MMS do any harm to red blood cells?

Q: I have an inherited Blood Disease "Beta Thalassemia Minor" in which my red blood cells are smaller and odd shaped from normal red blood cells. This causes me to be Anemic and I will always be anemic. Could you please tell me if MMS will do any harm to the red blood cells? I would really like to try MMS because of back problems, and arthritis.

A: MMS does not harm red blood cells. It will probably help the disease as well as your back problems and arthritis.

Will MMS cancel out the effect of other medications I am taking?

Q: I have a blocked vertebral artery, and spinal stenosis. I am taking too many prescriptions, but the ones that I wonder about are the aggrenox for the blocked artery, the neurontin for neuropathy, the clonapan and voltaren for inflammation. Somewhere in the literature I have read that the MMS cancels out the effects of medications. What do I do in this case? I do not want a stroke, or inflammation of all the joints, but would still like to be able to take the MMS. Is there a safe way to do this?

A: I have not noticed or heard that MMS cancels out the effects of any medications.

I think MMS can help you but take it separately from your other medications allowing 2 or 3 hours in between. Start with 1 drop of MMS and then slowly increase but only after a few days.

Is the fact that MMS turns to sodium chloride harmful in any way?

Q: It has been stated that after a period of 12 hours, the MMS turns to table salt. Is this harmful for high blood pressure or heart problems?

A: MMS converts to approximately 10 ml of sodium chloride which is table salt, which is only about half the size of a match head. You could probably not taste it in a half glass of water and besides the idea that salt causes high blood pressure is just a fable of modern medicine.

Can MMS harm Red Blood Cells in an Anemic patient?

Q: I would really like to try MMS because of back problems and arthritis.

However I have an inherited Blood Disease "Beta Thalassemia Minor" in which my red blood cells are smaller and odd shaped from normal red blood cells. This causes me to be Anemic and I will always be anemic. Could you please tell me if MMS will do any harm to the red blood cells?

A: MMS does not harm red blood cells. Most likely, it will help the disease as well as your back problems and arthritis.

Does MMS Conflict with Other Drugs?

Q: Will there be a conflict if a person is also taking Coumadin, Lipitor or other RX including like leavaquin or cipro antibiotics?

A: If the person is taking some kind of drug, medicine just wait from 2 to 3 hours apart. MMS does not conflict with Medicines but do not take them at the same time.

Why Does MMS Cause Burping and Strange After Taste?

Q: There is a lot of positive effects happening with the MMS. I am currently at 12 drops twice a day and experiencing mild nausea but burping what tastes like blood for a couple hours. I am taking the drops after eating. So my question is can MMS cause ulcers or stomach problems? Any other thoughts you have that my help my road to wellness would be appreciated. Thank You for all you have done to help humanity.

A: MMS has never caused stomach problems so far, and certainly not ulcers. However, it does kill growths in the stomach and other colonies of microorganisms. This could be the cause of the taste of blood, but it is only something that needs to be killed as MMS cannot kill beneficial organisms or healthy cells. Taking MMS is often killing microorganisms or larger organisms that are not causing problems in the present, but that will cause problems 10 or 20 years down the road. MMS has no food value at all to cause any kind of problem. It cannot kill beneficial body parts or organisms as it is a very weak oxidizer.

Blood Brain Barrier

Does MMS cross the blood/brain barrier to pull heavy lead or mercury out of the brain?

Q: Does MMS cross the blood/brain barrier to pull heavy lead or mercury out of the brain? I already ordered your product. I am just making sure that I fully treat my metal toxicity.

A: There is evidence to indicate that MMS crosses the barrier.

Bone Conditions

Will MMS slow down lung metastases associated with osteosarcoma?

Q: I have a unique case of lung metastases associated with osteosarcoma. I only have a few spots on my lungs and standard chemo/surgery will only extend my life by a few months. So while I am healthy I will try a few ideas. Will MMS slow things down as the metastasis is aggressive?

A: Yes it should help cure you. Just start with 1 to 2 drops and increase the dose by one or two drops per day.

Is it possible that the MMS is healing Osteoporosis and

Thyrotoxicosis?

Q: I have some questions about following disease: Osteoporosis, Thyrotoxicosis (Hashimoto-Thyreoiditis). Is it possible that the MMS is healing these diseases?

A: For osteoporosis once you start taking MMS be sure to get a high dose of calcium magnesium citrate in the liquid form for most health food stores. For Thyrotoxycosis chanced are that it would help do not know but it generally does and as far as autoimmune-disease MMS has help a lot of people with that disease.

Will MMS work on Hep C, Thrombocytopenia, Leukytosis, Crohn's Disease, Ankylosing Spondolitis, Osteopenia, Chronic severe Insomnia and Inflammatory, Rheumatoid, Degenerative and Osteoarthritis?

Q: I have Hep C, Thrombocytopenia, Leukytosis, Crohn's Disease, Ankylosing Spondolitis, Osteopenia, Chronic severe Insomnia and Inflammatory, Rheumatoid, Degenerative and Osteoarthritis. Will I be able to use this product safely?

A: Yes you will be able to use MMS safely if you follow the protocol starting off with 1/2 drop of MMS. Go to one of my sites listed below and follow the standard protocol, but be very slow to go to each new increase of MMS. Remember, when you feel sick, just lower the dose a few drops. MMS will help you with many of your diseases.

Brain Disorders

ALS, Alzheimer's, and others not yet reported on?

Q: ALS, Alzheimer's, and others not yet reported on?

A: There are a number of diseases that no one has called or emailed about so far. I cannot say much about these diseases as there are no reports, but if anyone does have a report I would certainly appreciate receiving it as thousands are waiting on these reports. Just send me a letter giving your experiences. You see MMS is different concerning reports. When I receive several reports giving success from different parts of the country I can start to believe the reports as these people could not all be working together to fool us, and we know that MMS does not cause harm.

What's the protocol to treat autism in a two year old kid?

Q: My Grand-Son has Autism! Can MMS help and if so what directions do you advise in terms of how much to take and how often. He is two years old.

A: Some have been helped. Start at 1/2 drop and work up to 3 drops for each 25 pounds. Go slow, increase drops one at a time.

Can MMS help my son who has autism?

Q: I have an 8 year old son with autism and he really is what you would call a "gut kid". I have done every good thing for him (gentle and alternative and diet) for 6 years but he still has

114

metabolic acidosis, a leaky gut, gut and brain inflammation. I would like to know if you have some specific stories about autistic kids doing well with MMS. You said that vinegar feeds yeast…and fermented food. But there is a very successful diet plan where fermented food and young coconut kefir are very healing and help cure yeast issues, did I misunderstand?

A: I really would appreciate it if you would read my book. Vinegar feeds Candida. Have all the coconut kefir you want. We used hair root analysis for heavy metal determinations. It seems to be fairly accurate. MMS is an oxidizer but different from any other oxidizers. The boy, I mentioned, is now doing a lot better. That is all I meant and all I said. He's still doing better. There are at least a thousand people who would like me to tell them what the book says, and I try, but I simply do not have the time. In my opinion it would help your son.

Do you have any data or information on the use of MMS and the cure of Alzheimer's?

Q: Do you have any data or information on the use of MMS and the cure of Alzheimer's?

A: I have known of people with Alzheimer's use MMS and they say they feel much better, I do not know if it cures it.

Does MMS remove heavy metals from the body? How safe and effective is it on children with Autism?

Q: Do you know where I can find information regarding MMS removing heavy metals from the body? Also, Does this cross the blood brain barrier? How safe is it for children? How effective is it on children with Autism?

A: I have had several phone calls where people have said MMS helped their children with autism. I personally had people tested for heavy metal before and after taking MMS and the heavy metals where almost reduced or totally reduced after 2 weeks. I do not know of any articles. There might be some but I do not know of any. Most of the people that are using the MMS are ordinary people and they do not write articles. Yes, it kills malaria in the brain and any number of reports of various different diseases of the brain, so there is no doubt that it crosses the blood brain barrier. Children have been taking MMS for the past 8 years.

Could you help me with suggestions concerning dosages and usage of the MMS and water combo package for maximum benefit?

Q: I would be grateful for your suggestions concerning dosages/usage of the MMS and the water combo package with the Prill beads & balls for maximum benefit:

Person #1 is recovering from breast cancer, is a smoker, and has undergone chemo: Person #2 is paraplegic with chronic bladder/kidney infections [also ordered colloidal silver for him], asthma and allergies, anxiety attacks and chronic depression, suspected add or onset of bipolar disorder: Person #3 is type 2 diabetic, high blood pressure, high cholesterol, degenerative arthritic condition, chronic obesity.

A: All these people you mention should follow the standard protocol for MMS. Start with two drops MMS, add ten drops of lemon or lime or citric acid solution as described in my book, mix, allow to set three minutes, add 1/2 glass or water and drink. Go the three drops, then to four, and then to 5. each time always using the correct amount of lemon or lime or citric. If nausea occurs, take a drop or two less next time. Then keep increasing the drops until you have reached 15 drops a day for 5 or 6 days then increase to three 15 drop doses a day until the problem is gone. Do not remain at three 15 drop doses a day for longer than 2 months. Reduce the amount as soon as possible. Then decrease to 4 to 6 drops a day for maintenance.

Cancer

Is it helpful to continue MMS if my carcinoma has not disappeared?

Q: I have been cleaning my mouth twice a day, and completed a week of 15 drops 3 X a day and applied the DMSO/MMS mix to my growth on the nose. It burned & tingled every time (repeated applications daily), and after about five days I stopped. The growth on my nose continued to grow back. Here is some more information about my health: I have been treated by the Bicom (measures frequency patterns) a few times recently and through this energetic testing the vials representing tumor, encephalon, skin, fibroma and melanoma resonated with me (my organs and tissue). The MMS tested very positively for me with the bicom. Here are my questions for you:

Considering how long I have been taking MMS, is it helpful to continue? Started end of April, quickly increased to 15 drops 2X day then on May 4th - 10th, 15 drops 3 X per day (one week). I have reverted back to 15 drops 2X per day.

The biopsy taken in late April said "invasive squamous cell carcinoma", the Bicom indicates melanoma. The surgeon believes the growth should be dug out and the area repaired asap. My own beliefs are challenged by this, but having this big thing on my nose is troublesome. I have some feelers out for someone to hear me out on this. I liked all the info on the MMS, and need a little information on the time-line and what other therapies are contradictory to the MMS.

The emotional burden for me has been great, and I feel like I have been dragging my feet to allow the MMS time to do the work....of undoing the poison in my body. I doubt myself and am afraid to share with people close to me for fear of their criticism and perceived stupidity on my part in dealing with this health issue. I have insurance but it is minimal, I am trying not to make decisions based on money. The dental work is still on the credit cards and there is some pressure there. I work as a caregiver, and am down to 18 hours a week, though I have to say the distraction of some work, from my own woes has been mostly good.

A: You have not been on MMS very long. It takes a lot longer. I would start to worry after two more months. There is one thing that I have some faith in and that is something called Aqualyte. It has some things in it that the body needs. You can get it at www.fredkaufman.com. It's cheap. It's has cured a lot of cancer all by itself, but it should work extra well with MMS as it has many things the body needs.

Surgeons have a 2.3% success rate. You have better chance hiding under your bed. All of the people that have died after coming here all died from the medical treatments. None of them died for cancer. I do not think therapies are contradictory to MMS as MMS only kills pathogens. It does not heal or anything. It kills pathogens. Fifteen drops three times a day is a good idea as long as it is not making you sick. Keep it up. If the taste gets really bad, find a strong grape juice or use extra lemon juice or citric acid after you ad the juice.

They have frozen grape juice is concentrated. That works pretty well.

I would like to know what protocol would be ideal for skin cancer; can I increase the dose or repetitions?

Q: I have been using MMS for a month, with 15 drops X 2 per day. I would like to know what protocol would be ideal for skin cancer; can I increase the dose or repetitions? I also have fungus. I have tried to buy the book with a discussion of cancer on line today but found it is not yet printed.

A: I am surprised that your skin cancer is not gone by now. Are you adding the citric acid or lemon juice drops? Here is something else that worked for me: Use DMSO mixed with 50% MMS topically on the cancer. Make a mixture of 6 drops of MMS and 30 drops of citric acid, wait 3 minutes, then take about 6 drops of that mixture and mix it with 6 drops of DMSO and apply that to the cancer. It should burn, and kill the cancer. The cancer should come off in next day or two.

Do you have any data about skin-cancer and MMS?

119

Q: I have a question for you. Maybe you can offer me some advice: My mother found a black spot on her shoulder, and the dermatologist is unsure what it is, so he wants to cut it out. It will leave a big scar, he said. Do you have any data about skin-cancer and MMS?

A: Yes, there is a lot of data on skin cancer and MMS. Normally it takes two to three weeks for MMS to eliminate cancers of the skin (melanomas). Do not let that dermatologist cut under any circumstances. I have heard so many horror stories about cutting. If it is not cancer, there might not be a problem, but if it is, most of the time it spreads when cut. Older people get black spots and that sort of thing, if it is not cancer, there is nothing to worry. Just take the MMS. If it is cancer, it will clear it up. If it is not cancer most likely there will be no change, but in either case, she is putting her life on the line to have it cut on. Cancer is spread by cutting. Medical people are often good people and they do try. But sometimes they are so out of it, they have no clue. When they cut and it spreads, they say well we are slowing it down. More people die from going to doctors than any other cause. Just take the MMS.

How long does citric acid last if refrigerated? Should I continue using it for the mixture if it's making me feel dizzy?

Q: When I took the MMS awhile back I was ok with the lemon juice activator but as soon as I took the citric acid I felt like I was poisoned and was very dizzy. I was only at about 5 drops twice a day. I cut back but could not shake the dizziness even at one drop with the citric acid. It has been a few weeks and I am about to try it again. I just threw out the citric acid because I read that it is perishable and should be kept refrigerated. I am now going to keep it refrigerated. My question is how long can it be kept refrigerated? My other question is if I possibly mixed it incorrectly could that because it to give a bad reaction such as mine? I mixed it as directed on the bag, 2 teaspoons of citric acid, to 3 ounces of distilled water. If the water is not exact as it may be off a little because there is no 1 or 3 ounce. measurements on my measuring cup, could that possibly be a problem? Well I am trying again tonight with 1 drop. I would greatly appreciate your response as I have breast cancer. I just had surgery and not sure yet what follow up treatment I will have, but would definitely like to try this possibly in conjunction.

A: If you are OK with lemon juice do not take citric acid. People who are allergic to citric acid should not take it, same as people who are allergic to vinegar. Citric acid will last indefinitely in the refrigerator, but do not use it. The amount of water that you take is not significant, but 4 ounces to 8 ounces would be better.

What do you recommend for a Leukemia patient who is experiencing the effects of MMS?

Q: A month ago a good friend was told he had acute Leukemia and that there was nothing the doctors good do for him. They gave him a minimum of three weeks and max of three months to live. He became very weak within 2 weeks, Then they gave him a blood transfusion and he felt much better for a few weeks but then got very weak again. It was at this point that I introduced him to your MMS. He was very interested and started on it a few days later.

I started him on 1 drop and increased by 1 drop per day. Yesterday July 9 he was up to 6 drops which he took 1 hour after breakfast and another 6 drops an hour later. After this second dose he had a lot of discomfort in his stomach. After a few hours of this he called me to come over and he was in great discomfort. I gave him a 500mg vitamin C with a glass of water and stayed with him for a while and he started to feel better and I left. A few hours later his wife called that he was very uncomfortable again, I went back and suggested he takes another vitamin C and to drink a lot of water. I went back to see him in the evening and he still had a lot of stomach discomfort, after several bowel movements and lots of water his wife also gave him tums (ant acid) with some Sprite.

She called me this morning to ask what to do now, he was very weak and still had stomach discomfort but was better than the day before. I am at a loss as to know what to recommend. It is now 23 hours since he took the last 6 drops of MMS with 30 drops of Citric Acid with 4 ounce of a juice blend of Apple, Grape, Pomegranate, and Citric Acid. There is 0 vitamin C and no indication of how much Citric Acid. According to your information it should all be neutralized by now.

I am afraid that in his condition with his blood in a much weakened state that he is not able to cope with the MMS upsetting his stomach.

What can you suggest I tell him? Should I tell him to stop the treatment for a few days? I feel bad that my first case has to be such a desperate situation and ma sorry I have to intrude in your already heavy work load, But I just need some help and desperately want this to turn into a success story.

A: My rule is, if it is making you sick, you are taking too much. I would drop back to one drop a dose. If he can take that without getting sick, wait 5 or 6 hours and then take two drops. If he feels sick, go back to one drop. Then go a second time with one drop and then try to increase again. Keep MMS going into him as much as possible by giving him up to 5 doses a day, but without making him sick. Five tiny doses is much better than one large dose. The pain in his stomach is undoubtedly something in there that needs to be killed. But do it slowly as to not make him sick.

If I give 2 cancer patients 15 drops right away, will it develop nausea?

Q: Mr. Kasumba is treating two cancer patients, but his recurring problem is if he goes ahead and gives them 15 drops right away they will develop nausea and other problems. I remember your teaching in book 2 that the worse a patient is the less they can tolerate a strong dose in one go. Do you start even very sick patients off with two drops and increase slowly in such cases? Another one: You recommend avoiding nausea that a patient can take the MMS after a meal. In such a case, will that not influence its efficiency, if the patient has eaten calcium rich food and that food gets mixed with the MMS drink?

A: The only person that should start out at 15 drops is one with malaria. Then wait an hour and use a second 15 drop dose. (Always activated with 5 drops of lemon juice or citric acid solution for each MMS drop. Wait 3 minutes and add 1/2 to one glass of water or juice.) All other persons should start out at 1 or 2 drops. For healthy persons, increase as quickly as possible. For sick persons increase a little more slowly but not much. For cancer patients the same is true. Back off when they get sick, or have diarrhea.

My husband took 12 drops and had some reactions, have you heard of these reactions?

Q: My husband and I were at 15 drops once daily before he left on a trip. He missed a few days and then resumed at 6 or 8 drops a day. I had informed him of the importance of a slow and gradual buildup to 15 drops. Unfortunately, he decided to jump to 12 drops/twice daily from 6. Yesterday evening after his second 12-drop dose of the day, he felt nauseous. We tried apples, peppermint….nothing helped. I was quite concerned as he went through about three rounds of vomiting, multiple times during each round (during a 2-2.5 hr span of time). In total, he probably vomited 9 or 10 times. The MMS was ingested about 1.5-2 hrs after a meal. He is just getting over a cold. Have you ever heard of such a reaction? We are unaware of any illness that might bring on such a strong reaction. She is thrilled as her husband's PSA levels have increased again. He has undergone various treatments for prostate cancer.

A: Many people get that kind of reaction. It was coming. It is not something that he caused by going from 6 to 12 drops although that brought it on faster. He's just been digging the microorganisms out from deep in this body. He will be better now. However, if the apples do not work, try 5000 mg of vitamin C in a glass of water. PSA levels often increase a little before beginning to decrease, however, more prostate cancer cured so far than anything else.

What is the recommended dose for treating extra nodal cutaneous lymphoma?

Q: I have extra nodal cutaneous lymphoma. I have a tumor on my breast that is 1 1/2 inches in diameter. It grew from 3/4 inch in about six months. I have been taking MMS since September 2007 six drops twice a day. The tumor got bigger since then. A friend told me to ask you what amount do I need to take to get results. I have been under treatment with a holistic doctor who uses the Voll machine to check all my organs and general health. I have been doing nosodes from Germany. These nosodes were to detox me from all kinds of metals, lead, mercury. Also for pesticides, arsenic and strychnine and other poisons. I was diagnosed in 2002 and have been in remission twice. This is the first time since 2002 that the tumor on my breast started growing.

Please let me know what you recommend on the amount of MMS I should take daily.

The only medicines I am on is an enzyme called Wobenzym am taking 4 3x a day and also Paw Cell reg 4 a day. If you have any other suggestions I am open to them. I really do not want to have surgery but right now that may be my only choice. Thank you again for your time and input.

A: The basic overlying principle is if you are not getting well, you are not taking enough. I do not believe 6 drops a dose is enough to treat cancer unless you are using it numerous times during a day. If you use strong grape juice (that does not have vitamin C added) the taste will not be so bad. One should maintain enough going in to keep one just below the nausea level. So this is what I would tell someone if there were talking to me about a similar case. Drink plenty of water to wash out the poisons from the dead cancerous tissues. That should keep you going to the bathroom often.

I keep trying to not prescribe but it's hard to do that and also help. When the time comes they probably would not care what I say or did anyway. Follow the protocol and you will probably do very good. Everyone else does.

What is the next step after taking 15 drop 2 times a day?

Q: I have been taking MMS since 3/2/08 on the advice of Ed Heft. I had major surgery to remove my kidney, ureter, and part of my bladder BEFORE I was told by our esteemed medical community that I was going to die from cancer anyway. Luckily, the first cancer doctor was honest enough to tell me that my transitional cell carcinoma would not respond to chemo or radiation therapy. We then began an intensive search to find alternative treatments, and were very fortunate to find Ed Heft. I have been working very hard to become healthy, and fully expect to beat the cancer. I have changed my diet as recommended, use one of Ed's BL's daily, flush my liver every two weeks, have a new found spirituality, and have been using UREA mixture & MMS daily. I am much healthier then I was before my cancer diagnosis. My question regarding MMS is just some clarification, and maybe as little guidance. Since I used all of my allotted leave of absence from my job to be gutted by the medical industry, I have been working full time in my job as a HVAC wholesale salesman. This job requires me to drive 600-800 miles per week. Ed counseled me to try using MMS only in the evenings during the work week and try to increase it over the weekends while I was stationary. I started with 1 drop dose, and over a 6 week period I was up to 15 drops 1X/day. The MMS website says for cancer I need to get to 15 drops 3X a day for at least a week, and then a maintenance dose thereafter. After a couple weeks @ 15 drops 1X/day, I tried to increase it to 2X a day, and had no problem with nausea or diarrhea for a few days, so I stupidly tried to increase it to 3X a day. This gave me a terrible case of diarrhea, and you may remember I called you on the phone to discuss how to proceed. You recommended that I try to split the dose up to 5 drops 3X/day, and build from there. Due to the traveling, and sometime overnight stays involved with my work, that is just about impossible to manage. I have to keep it from direct light, and have fresh fruit acid to activate it, and keep it in my hot car. Consequently, I am doing still just doing 15 drops 1X/day, every day. Other than the taste beginning to get to me, I am noticing no real effects. I have consumed about 1/3 of the bottle of MMS. My question is how to continue using the MMS. Should I just do what I am doing till the bottle is empty? That should take about a year total at this rate. I could possibly try it 2X a day for awhile, but my treatment management with food juicing, fresh fruits & veggies to eat, liver flushes, and UREA mixtures, I am having difficulty maintaining it all. The long process of building up the dosage 2X/day will tax my schedule and processes. Do you think it's possible that I could have achieved some level of improvement that would allow me to go to a weekly maintenance dosage? In late April, I had my 90 day follow up medical tests, and the butchers say I do not have cancer in me right now. The OSU

(That's right, THE OHIO STATE MEDICAL CENTER) had a previous blood test for me from 10 years ago, which showed on the report, and all my major indicators are better now than they were back then. I am 45 years old. Would I take an older persons maintenance dose, or a younger person's dose? Please let me know your thoughts on this. My phone numbers are listed below if you wish to discuss farther.

A: Keep in mind, the MMS has no food value at all. It only kills things. If the cancer is gone, I would revert to older person maintenance of 6 drops a day and let it go at that. Eventually you will want to go back and do the 15 drops three times a day, but it does not seem like that is productive at this time.

What dose should I give a patient with a Tumor in his left lung?

Q: I have a dear customer I need assistance with. He has a tumor in his left lung. He is starting his MMS protocol today. I recommended that he do 1-2 drops 3 times/day. I have explained all of the information about taking MMS at least 2 hours away from other supplements, medicines and also to do so, on an empty stomach. Could you please give us more direction on how fast he should go? I believe he is in his late 60's or older and in very active with tennis. I have copied him on this e-mail and you are most welcome to communicate with him directly.

A: Just go as fast as you can in increasing the number of times per day and the amount per day, but the minute you feel some nausea coming on, back off, not stopping, but taking less for a while and then begin to increase again. Do not back off more than one day and continue always striving to take more without getting nauseous. The nausea is of course coming from the dead cells or viruses. Some people's bodies can get rid of the poison faster than others. Fresh apples, as much as two after taking a dose of MMS will absorb poisons, so does clay, and so does charcoal, or just use the apples. Keep it up. Many people have said they are well after having tumors in the lungs.

Can one overcome cancer with MMS?

Q: Overcoming Cancer?

A: Many people have called me up to say that their cancer is gone after taking MMS. I have emails and telephone calls from people who the doctors gave 2 weeks left to live. Of all of those who called me, they are all back working now. On rare occasions, the people do not seem to respond very well, but no one has ever sent an email or phone call to say that after someone started taking MMS, that he had died. It has probably happened, but for the most part, people improved or got well.

What's the protocol for tumors in lungs?

Q: I have a dear customer I need assistance with. He has a tumor in his left lung.

A: I recommended that he does 1-2 drops 3 times/day. I have explained all of the information about taking MMS at least 2 hours before or after other supplements and medicines.

Will MMS help me with biliary cirrhosis, melanoma on

129

my leg and other numerous physical injuries?

Q: I have massive health problems–congenitally defective kidneys which over the years have caused biliary cirrhosis of the liver–the later I have had for at least twenty years–ten years ago I almost died from brain cancer-and a melanoma on my leg–a woman from Denmark turned up in my life and saved it– but generally my life has been one long nightmare–besides all the sickness–major physical injuries too numerous to mention-i just wonder what you think–my reactions seem outside anything you talk about.

A: Use lemon or lime juice instead of vinegar. Your reactions seem reasonable considering your condition, you should just continue with the MMS.

Will MMS help a 78 year old woman with breast cancer that has metastasized to her lungs?

Q: My mom has breast cancer that has metastasized to her lungs. She is on chemo and also on a very involved holistic program that I devised after reading a lot of material and taking into consideration what she can and cannot do. She is 78 and cannot swallow pills. I am impressed by your MMS and am wondering what you feel the best method is to try this. Should she start out with one drop a day – add the acidic (wait 3 minutes) and apple juice (without vitamin C added) then drink and then up it if she feels okay. Do you feel this will help cure her cancer and if so what kinds of signs should we look for?

A: I think it will help. You are right about starting with 1 drop.

How effective is MMS for cancer?

Q: My daughter has cancer. How effective is it for cancer ? My daughter is scared about anything except her chemo. I want to help her but I do not want to make her worse. What do you think ?

A: MMS has been successful with hundreds of cancer cases. There is no evidence that chemo helps. They get excited when they increase the life expectancy by two months. Read their evidence closely. There has never been any real evidence that proves chemotherapy helps cure cancer. Yes, they have some improvements or remissions, but those who refuse chemo have the same remission and improvements. The fact is: those who refuse the chemo suffer less and live longer. MMS on the other hand can give 40 years longer rather than 2 months.

What type of water should I use to add it to the activated MMS?

Q: I am beginning to share about the MMS with many people and I want to be very clear about this water issue because I am hearing different stories. I have my own water filter and have been using my filtered water to make both the citric acid solution (1 teaspoon crystals to 9 teaspoon filtered water) and then using my filtered water to add to the activated solution for drinking. Is what I am doing okay or am I only to be using distilled water for the citric solution and for the drinking... is the filtered water okay for the drink part that I am adding to the other? Please clarify. I have a woman to talk to later this week who has been diagnosed with leukemia and I want to be giving her the correct information.

A: Really, the water is not an issue. Use distilled water, or tap water, or bottled water, or river water. The MMS is a killer. It kills all the bad stuff in the water. The amount of minerals that you will get from a dose of MMS even from tap water is not enough to hurt anything. If you want to be perfect, used distilled water. Some people do not like distilled water, but that amount of distilled water will not hurt the most sensitive person.

Do the side effects of MMS mean that it's not working on my cancer?

Q: I am on a protocol alternating MMS with Vitamin C. I started MMS last Saturday and followed your advice to start with 2 drops and I am upping the ante until I hit 15 drops. The first few days went ok, but as the dosage increased I start getting more nauseous with each dose. I am up to 11 drops and am getting too sick to take the second dose. Last night I tossed and turned all night with stomach cramps and a headache. Is this unusual and should I either discontinue or change my dosage? I desperately want the MMS to destroy the cancer, but because of the uncomfortable side effects am wondering if the MMS is actually worsening the problem.

A: When you begin to feel bad, reduce the number of drops you are taking. Always back off and take less drops. I say that because if people continue on the same vein, they begin to question if it is helping or worsening. So please back off until you are not feeling bad. Remain at that level of drops for two or three days and then begin increasing slowly. Increase one added drop for a day or two and keep increasing until you begin feeling a little nauseous then back off. Do not allow yourself to feel bad. Back off instead, but keep pushing. Increase as much as you can without feeling bad.

Does MMS work on advanced stages of cancer?

Q: My friend has become chemo, on one place in her head, the question is can she still take the MMS without the MMS neutralize the effect of the chemo??

She is taking now about 4 times a day 4 drops without becoming sick, her test of the blood where negative even higher....so does this mean that the MMS does not work for her advance stage?? She tolerates no higher amounts in this moment.

A: They cannot show you any evidence that chemo helps. Why take it? Hundreds of cancer patients have written or called saying they have had help or completely recovered with MMS. I do not know what the blood tests were but if it was worse it was not from the MMS. It had to be from the chemo. I suggest the AMAS test. If you really want to check MMS out, go to my web site; there, you can get all the information about the cancer AMAS test that anyone can buy and is 99% effective. Doctors do not use it because they do not make any money from it. But anyone can take the test, use MMS for a couple of weeks and take the test again. It immediately tells if there has been an improvement.

What can I use instead of lemon juice or any beverage with vitamin C?

Q: My brother has prostate cancer and we are wanting to use

MMS. Questions:

He has a reaction of canker sores when he gets Vitamin C in his system. We started out with 1 drop in lemon juice, added 1/3 C cranberry juice (no sugar or vitamin C additives). We did that twice the first day and Bob has broken out with a canker sore. We are pretty sure it's due to the lemon and cranberry juice. We are afraid to continue as he will end up with a mouth full of sores and plays trumpet for a living. Would you have a suggestion? Also, my sister-in-law wanted to use MMS for maintenance. She ended up with terrible heartburn using the same mixture as above. Would you have some thoughts on that situation?

A: Well in his case, I would suggest using vinegar in place of the lemon juice and then try 1 drop once a day. All those allergies are simply bad bacteria somewhere in the system. Once they are killed off, no allergies. But it might take a while. Just work at slowly increasing the drops. All prostate cancer cases have been successful at getting rid of the cancer so far, that is what they have said. I only take their word for it.

My wife is suffering from an aggressive metastatic breast cancer. Is MMS likely to be a solution?

Q: My wife is suffering from an aggressive metastatic breast cancer. Is MMS likely to be a solution?

A: MMS has helped a lot of people and it can be a solution. If she is taking any other medicine, drug wait from 3 to 4 hours apart.

Can I safely give my son with Leukemia the MMS alongside the chemo pills?

Q: My teenage son is in remission from an acute leukemia and is on daily chemotherapy pills. Can I safely give him the MMS alongside the chemo pills?

A: I have had no one indicate a problem between and MMS and chemotherapy pills. There have been many who have indicated that they were doing both, but the fact that they never mentioned a problem does not mean that one does not exist. I do not know of a problem. Chemo tears your immune system down. There is no evidence that they can show you that indicates that chemo has ever prolonged anyone's life. However, there is a great deal of evidence that chemo has destroyed immune systems. The MMS builds the immune system up. Chemo tears it down. Hopefully you wind up with no damage done.

If there was any logic in it one would ask for actual evidence where chemo has made someone live longer, like, this group had cancer and they took chemo and they lived longer than this group over here with a similar cancer who did not take chemo. But no such evidence exists. So they just give a lot of informative double talk that sounds official, but proves nothing.

Will MMS slow down lung metastases associated with osteosarcoma?

Q: I have a unique case of lung metastases associated with osteosarcoma. I only have a few spots on my lungs and

135

standard chemo/surgery will only extend my life by a few months. So while I am healthy I will try a few ideas. Will MMS slow things down as the metastasis is aggressive?

A: Yes it should help cure you. Just start with 1 to 2 drops and increase the dose by one or two drops per day.

Is there any cases known that it helps Parkinson's or if not do you feel that it can help?

Q: My husband has bladder cancer and diverticulitis. I have Parkinson's disease. We have both been taking MMS for a couple of months now. I have ordered your book. I know that MMS helps cancer however is there any cases known that it helps Parkinson's or if not do you feel that it can help?

A: I had several people that told me MMS has helped them with Parkinson, I think it will help but no one has told me that they have been cured yet. I believe that it may be necessary to take MMS by IV infusion or enemas to make a big difference. I have good reports for a lot of disease that they are reporting and many are being cured but none that I am aware of for Parkinson's disease.

Would MMS help my wife with an aggressive metastatic breast cancer?

Q: My wife is suffering from an aggressive metastatic breast cancer. Is MMS likely to be a solution?

A: MMS has helped a lot of people and it can be a solution. If she is taking any other medicine, drug wait from 3 to 4 hours apart.

Is it OK to take 30 to 45 drops of MMS for treating prostate cancer?

Q: I have prostate cancer which has spread to my bones. I have been taking 30 to 45 drops of MMS for a few weeks and have not felt any difference. Maybe I have not given it enough time? I am going to increase to 60 drops today do you have any suggestions? I just started the Indian herb is that ok with MMS provided they are 4 hours apart?

A: It is ok to take the Indian herb 4 hours apart from MMS. I do not think that you are adding the citric or lemon acid and waiting 3 minutes. You cannot possibly be using the activator. You need to begin using the lemon, lime, or citric acid and wait three minutes and add water or juice. I would also suggest you drop back to about 8 or 10 drops or so. There is no way you could be doing things right and be taking 45 drops with activation. It would knock you out.

Is it OK to take MMS while on chemo tablets?

Q: I have been on tablet form of chemo called Xeloda taking 4x 500mg tablets twice daily. I have just started to take MMS drops and I am wondering if this is okay to take while on chemo tablets?

A: Well, you can do chemo and MMS and it will not hurt anything, but chemo destroys the immune system and MMS builds it up. If one of them cancels out the other, you are at zero. Go to the site www.lifeone.org and click on "You have nothing to fear from cancer." Then realize that AMAS is a 99% effective cancer test that has been around for more than 25 years. You can buy a test on the internet for $165 from www.oncolabinc.com MMS is better than the cure that they are selling, but the data is fantastic. So use MMS for a while and then use this test to prove it is working.

What are your suggestions for a cancer patient who cannot get past five drops of MMS?

Q: My friend has done a lot off chemo and has tumors in her belly as well in her head, so it's a very serious condition, she can handle now 2 times a day 4 drops, we are trying now if she can tolerate every hour 3 drops.... Normally when she comes up to 5 drops she gets nausea and has to vomit. What do you think?

A: Go to the site www.lifeone.org and click on "You have nothing to fear from cancer." Then realize that AMAS is a 99% effective cancer test that has been around for more than 25 years. You can buy a test on the internet for $165 from www.oncolabinc.com MMS is better than the cure that they are selling, but the data is fantastic. So use MMS for a while and then use this test to prove it is working.

Would starting at 5 drops of MMS and then increasing it to 15 drops be a good protocol against breast cancer?

Q: I was diagnosed with Breast Cancer 6 years ago. The cancer came back in my liver, lungs and bones. I did 22 rounds of chemotherapy. I made it through that (finished chemotherapy on June of 2006) and I am holding pretty stable. I started taking MMS on Oct 10th. 1st Dose 10am 5 drops MMS, 25 drops citric acid 3 min. Wait added 1/2 glass fresh pineapple juice, and increased the dose up to 15 drops. Does this seems like a good protocol for someone with Breast Cancer and do you have anyone else that has a good idea how much it will take and length of time?

A: That seems like a very good protocol. MMS is usually very fast in that the body heals very fast after the item is destroyed. Expect anywhere from 2 weeks to 2 months to overcome the cancer. If there is a possibility of checking the cancer without invasive methods would be good to do after two weeks. Each case is different. I do not know anyone who would give out suggestions at this time.

Is it all right to keep using the MMS and to gradually increase the dosage now that I started chemotherapy due to Type T Lymphoma?

Q: I am suffering from Type T lymphoma right now and I am going through Chemo Therapy Treatment. I was taking the MMS up to 7 drops twice daily before the chemo started. Is it all right to keep using the MMS and to gradually increase the dosage at this time?

A: Yes keep on taking MMS and continue increasing the dose just wait from 3 to 4 hours after Chemo Therapy Treatment before taking MMS, I would prefer for you to stop taking chemo, but that is up to you.

Why did a cotton ball soaked with MMS leave a mark on my skin?

Q: I have metastatic bone cancer & have begun taking MMS. I also have a large tumor up near my collarbone. I tried 2 drops MMS diluted with 1/4 teaspoon fresh lemon juice & soaked a cotton wool ball with the solution, which I then taped onto the tumor & left it for approx. 2 hours. I did feel a burning stinging sensation & when I removed the cotton ball, it had burnt my skin, leaving a red mark. Did I do something wrong?

A: Yes, you cannot leave MMS on the skin for more than 3 minutes you must wash it off.

Is it all right to keep using the MMS and to gradually increase the dosage now that I am having chemotherapy?

Q: I am suffering from Type T lymphoma right now and I am going through chemotherapy treatment. I was taking the MMS up to 7 drops twice daily before the chemo started. Is it all right to keep using the MMS and to gradually increase the dosage at this time?

A: Yes keep on taking MMS and continue increasing the dose just wait from 3 to 4 hours after chemo therapy treatment before taking MMS.

Does MMS help Parkinson's disease?

Q: My husband has bladder cancer and diverticulitis. I have Parkinson's disease. We have both been taking MMS for a couple of months now. I have ordered your book. I know that MMS helps cancer however is there any cases known that it helps Parkinson's or if not do you feel that it can help?

A: I had several people that told me MMS has helped them with Parkinson, I think it will help but no one has told me that they have been cured yet. I believe that it may be necessary to take MMS by IV infusion or enemas to make a big difference. I have good reports for a lot of disease that they are reporting and many are being cured but none that I am aware of for Parkinson's disease.

Would MMS help my wife who's suffering from an aggressive breast cancer that is resistant to chemotherapy?

Q: My wife is suffering from an aggressive breast cancer that is resistant to chemotherapy. Is MMS likely to be a solution? Is there a possible interaction with other drugs?

A: MMS has helped a lot of people and it can be a solution, if you go to my web page you can see a cancer protocol and use that also I have a list of suppliers of MMS. If she is taking other medication wait 3 to 4 hours before taking.

Can I use more than 25 drops in a sever case? Should it be used topically on a breast cancer lesion?

Q: The normal protocol is up to 25 drops in severe cases however, I am interested in knowing can one use more? And should it be used topically on a breast cancer lesion?

A: There have been people who took up to 75 drops for cancer on the throat so I would assume you can take the same amount for breast Cancer there has been no bad reports, however on the breast cancer with lesions I would suggest using the Indian herb because many people I know have used Indian heard on the breast or any wherein the body. The Indian herb has the ability to kill the cancer directly as apposed through the blood but you should take both.

How can I combine both MMS and Stabilized Oxygen for treating Breast Cancer?

Q: I have breast cancer that I have used the laser method as an alternative treatment. What type of dosage would you recommend for this since I am unsure of the status? Also I have a case of 2.33.ounce. Stabilized Oxygen from World Nutrition that I would like to utilize for this treatment. I called and asked the company if they did indeed use 3.5% sodium chlorite and they said they use 5.0%. How would that affect the number of drops I should use?

A: Use 5 drops for each 1 drop of recommended for MMS but use the same number of drops of citric acid which would mean equal Numbers use 5 drops citric acid for every 5 drops of stabilized oxygen.

Will MMS work for Multiple Sclerosis (MS), Breast cancer, Psoriasis or Eczema?

Q: I was wondering if MMS will work for Multiple Sclerosis and breast cancer. Has anybody written to you about using it for MS or after cancer maintenance? Have you found that it also works for Psoriasis or Eczema?

A: Several people who have MS have reported to me that they have overcome all or almost all of their symptoms and that they have their life back. I cannot promise you anything and I certainly would not say that I know for sure that it cures anything. But a hundred thousand people so far have reported being well or a lot better. If it stays cured I do not know. Not enough time has passed since the reports of those who said they are back to their life.

Carpal Tunnel Syndrome

Will MMS help with arthritis, inflammation in my foot and some pain in my hand that might be carpal tunnel syndrome?

Q: My daughter had me order some MMS. I have had horrible pain in my left hand, elbow and arm it could be carpal tunnel syndrome, but I have had that before and this just feels different. Will MMS help? I also found out that I have arthritis and inflammation in my foot can MMS help this? Can I use 100% cherry juice?

A: Yes. It will help you there have been good results for inflammation and arthritis. Just make sure the juice does not contain Vitamin C (ascorbic acid) then it is ok to use.

Chickenpox

I am experiencing what seems to be an outbreak of shingles on my back. Are you aware of anyone using any particular method of taking the MMS for this viral outbreak?

Q: I am experiencing what seems to be an outbreak of shingles on my back. Are you aware of anyone using any particular method of taking the MMS for this viral outbreak?

A: There is a lot of people taking MMS for shingles you should take it by mouth but also get a small spray bottle 2 ounce mix 20 drop of MMS and 100 drops of citric acid solution of lemon juice wait 3 minutes and fill the rest of the 2 ounce bottle with water, spray it on your back 2 or 3 times a day and keep taking MMS by mouth, MMS will cause it to break loose and it needs to come off.

By taking this product can one avoid getting shingles?

Q: By taking this product can one avoid getting shingles, because of a person's age and having had chicken pox as a child?

A: Yes, one can avoid getting shingles or chicken pox but if you do contract any of these diseases, what you can do is take MMS by mouth, but also get a small spray 2 ounce bottle mix 20 drops of MMS with 100 drops of citric acid solution, or lemon juice, wait 3 minutes and fill the rest of the 2 ounce bottle with water, spray it on 2 or 3 times a day and keep taking MMS by mouth.

Children

I have 2 orphans that are HIV positive, please let me know how to use MMS with them?

Q: I am a missionary in Mozambique caring for 40 orphans. 2 are HIV positive and dear to me. Please tell me more about how to use this medicine with them. One is a girl 6 years and the other a boy 9 years. I have also suffered too much with malaria last year and would like to take it for that. The directions for usage do not seem real clear to me. 2 drops each hour until all the 2 drops add up to 15? I am confused. I am also hopeful.

A: Well, yes, with HIV or AIDS start with one drop and increase each day one drop until you are at 3 drops for each 25 pounds of body weight. For malaria, you need to shock it. Use 15 drops of MMS and 75 drops of activator. Use lemon juice drops as the activator or vinegar or citric acid activator. Wait 1 or 2 hours and hit it with a second 15 drops dose, same as the first dose. That's all you will need. That kills the malaria.

What is the dosage for people with Malaria?

Q: The MMS just arrived here today. After I return from Alexandria in four or five days, I will start treating two people with malaria right here in Cairo. Sudanese nationals. Then in a week or so after that, I will head down to the border and treat a few people there. I will start out with 18 drops. If that makes them vomit then I will go down to 6 drops every hour for 4 hours, as you prescribed in your email below. How long does it take to clear the patient from malaria?

A: 90% of the cases of malaria will be free of malaria with all symptoms gone in 4 hours. It will look like miracles. You just have to do it right. Use 15 to 18 drops depending upon the person the bigger the person the more drops, but do not go over 18 drops for the first dose or under 15 for smaller persons. Then in one to 4 hours give the second dose. Normally the first dose cures the malaria and the second dose goes deeper to kill anything remaining. Remember, all doses require the lemon juice or citric acid, 5 drops for each 1 drop of MMS, wait three minutes and add the juice. I always use pineapple juice, about 1/2 glass and I often dilute the pineapple juice with 50% water to make it go further. Children use less. For malaria judge their size and weight but it should be 3 drops for each 25 pounds (11.4 kg) of body weight. When you have a long line of kids, you do not have time to weigh them. Just judge their weight. Just error on the side of too much MMS rather than too little. If only a few people vomit. Do not change the doses. Only change if most people are vomiting. Judge these things correctly as when other people see someone vomiting they will refuse to take MMS.

Would it be OK for a woman to work her way up to 15 drops if she has a 14 month old daughter who is still nursing?

Q: I do understand that a baby under 25 pounds should only take 2 drops of the MMS but my daughter is wondering if it will be ok after she gets past 2 drops and works her way up to 15 drops, if too much will come through the breast milk for her 14 month old daughter who is still nursing. The baby probably weighs about 25 pounds although I do not know her exact weight.

A: We have never had any problem with MMS coming through the breast milk. I doubt that it would, but it would be healthy if it did.

Since I am pregnant, Is the six drop dosage powerful enough to kill worms?

Q: I am breastfeeding my one-year-old child. A friend of my husband told us about your product MMS and wrote to you about whether it is safe to take while breastfeeding. You said it was safe, but to limit it to the 6 drop dosage. I believe I can feel parasites / worms moving around inside of me and have seen my waste moving around in the toilet. I think my two daughters may have parasites / worms too. On the bottle of MMS, it says that the 15 drop dosage should be used to kill parasites / worms. My questions are:

1. Is the six drop dosage powerful enough to kill the worms or should I be doing something else? Should I take a drug to kill the worms and then take your product? Also, is the child and baby dosages strong enough to kill the worms in the kids?

2. Can I take the 6 drop dosage and give the baby dosage to my one-year-old (breastfeeding) daughter at the same time?

3. My 5 year old daughter, husband, and I have been taking MMS for 4 days. We are up to 4 drops once a day, taking one extra drop each day. How many times a day should we be taking MMS?

A: Do not worry about 6 drops. Go for 15 to kill the worms, But go slowly working up to that does one drop at a time. You can take the MMS from one to three times a day. Look at how you feel and how much you think you can take without making yourself too nauseous. It is good for babies, but if the baby becomes nauseous you might have to use a bottle for a few days, not likely, but maybe. If the 3 drops for 25 pounds of body weight does not do it, use more.

What's the protocol to treat autism in a two year old kid?

Q: My Grand-Son has Autism! Can MMS help and if so what directions do you advise in terms of how much to take and how often. He is two years old.

A: Some have been helped. Start at 1/2 drop and work up to 3 drops for each 25 pounds. Go slow, increase drops one at a time.

Is MMS safe to take during pregnancy, especially during the initial trimester?

Q: I have only just started taking MMS & have discovered today that I am pregnant. Is MMS safe to take during pregnancy, especially during the initial trimester?

A: There has been good reports with MMS and pregnancy just start off with a low dose and increase slowly.

Is it safe for my pregnant wife to use MMS?

Q: I wonder if it is safe for my wife to use MMS. She is 6 months pregnant.

A: Yes it is safe to take MMS while being pregnant. Just start with small amounts.

Is MMS safe to take while pregnant?

Q: Is MMS is safe to take while pregnant?

A: Yes, just start with small amounts.

Will any of the heavy metal toxins that I have seeped into my breast milk? Is MMS harmful for my baby?

Q: I am a nursing mother and take MMS I have a lot of heavy metal toxins, parasites, and Lyme disease, will taking MMS hurt my baby or will any of the heavy metals that MMS is removing from my body seep into my breast milk?

A: MMS will not harm your baby MMS it does not seep into the breast milk it is OK take MMS wile breastfeeding. There is a lot of mothers taking MMS who are breastfeeding or pregnant and they have not reported anything bad back to us.

Cholesterol

Can MMS help with my cholesterol? Is it normal to feel tired for a while?

Q: I am 65 years old and have used Chemicals most of my life Lacquers and paints. I started using MMS about a week ago and feeling quite worn out most of the time since I started using the MMS I am using about 7 to 8 drops twice a day had a bad case of sitting on the toilet but only lasted for a few hours. I was wondering if it is normal to be tired for a while. Also can this stuff help with cholesterol?

A: It is normal to have diarrhea or vomiting that is a good indicator, also is normal for you to get tired, there are people who take it at night and they sleep really good and since you get tired you should drink it when going to sleep. Remember when you get diarrhea just lower the dosage and when it stops increase it.

Chronic Fatigue

Would MMS help the lyme if bartonella is also there?

Q: I am new to the lyme world. I was diagnosed with CFS and sick for 24 years. Now my 24 year old daughter is sick with lyme and bartonella or mycoplasma. (what I now know, I probably have lyme too.) Would MMS help the lyme if bartonella is also there?

And, right now she chose to start cumanda and samento before she goes on an antibiotic, would MMS fit into this regime?

One last question, if you would not mind, how does MMS differ from the Salt/C protocol?

My daughter is on DHEA and testosterone cream, midodrine due to low blood pressure (I am not sure if it is working) and salt tablets. She just started cumanda and samento because she is doing school 5 days a week and is afraid of herx from antibiotics since she is getting married in August and has Bar exam in July.

A: MMS is chlorine dioxide, an oxidizer that kills pathogens, but does not touch the rest of the body. It is totally different from the salt and vitamin C action. At this point I do not know anything that is guaranteed in handling lyme. MMS has proved effective depending upon the protocol and the person. It occurs to me that salt seems to drive the lyme out into the open, and the salt might work well with MMS. So the state of the lyme protocol is still being tested by many different people. But in my opinion, the best weapon so far is MMS and chemistry does not have a better weapon even in theory.

Do you have some cases in which patients with Chronic Fatigue were healed with MMS?

Q: My wife has chronic fatigue and my mother-in-law has multiple sclerosis. Do you have some cases that patients with this condition were healed with MMS?

A: I do have some success stories for chronic fatigue but I would have to ask people for permission in order to pass it around, for MS Several people who have MS have reported to me that they have overcome all or almost all of their symptoms and that they have their life back.

What is the protocol for taking MMS for Lyme disease and severe CFIDS?

Q: I have very severe CFIDS (chronic fatigue and immune dysfunction syndrome), and I am totally bedridden much of the time. Several doctors feel I may also have late stage Lyme disease as well as metals.

I did not tolerate 3 months of antibiotics at all. Can MMS help me? I started MMS treatment two nights ago. I put 2 drops in a cup, mixed 1/2 teaspoon of lime juice. Waited for 3 minutes. Added 1/3 cup of water. I want to make sure I am doing this right.

It seems like MMS also kills many bacteria. Can MMS eradicate viruses and bacteria that hide out in cells and replicate in ways that the immune system does not find them?

A: For every drop of MMS you need to add 5 drops of citric acid, lime or lemon juice, wait 3 minutes and then add half a glass of water or juice.

The most effective way that I have found to help eradicate Lyme disease so far is to take 3 or 4 drops, 3 or 4 times a day.

A lot of people who have Lyme disease have taken MMS and it seems to help quite a bit, but no one has reported back to me that they are completely cured yet.

I personally had people tested for heavy metals before and after taking MMS and the heavy metals were totally reduced after 2 weeks

Cirrhosis

Will MMS help me with biliary cirrhosis, melanoma on my leg and other numerous physical injuries?

Q: I have massive health problems–congenitally defective kidneys which over the years have caused biliary cirrhosis of the liver–the later I have had for at least twenty years–ten years ago I almost died from brain cancer-and a melanoma on my leg–a woman from Denmark turned up in my life and saved it–but generally my life has been one long nightmare–besides all the sickness–major physical injuries too numerous to mention-i just wonder what you think–my reactions seem outside anything you talk about.

A: Use lemon or lime juice instead of vinegar. Your reactions seem reasonable considering your condition, you should just continue with the MMS. Do not give up. Others who where having similar problems eventually came through. It may take a while.

Colds and Flu

My brother's wife has had a cold for a month, what protocol should she use?

Q: 1-the cold/flu I have had is affecting many people in my area(Montreal) my brother was lucky-only 2 days but his wife has had it for over 1 month now also chemtrails are bad-like a calcium dust that infiltrates into one's home. That cold/flu gets stuck in the bronchi and into your bones (pain). One needs at least 6 drops of MMS, 3 times per day to get rid of it- less drops will not do it. My MMS limit is 6 drops 3 times per day MMS got rid of that cold/flu within 7 days or so.

A: Make up a 20 drop dose in about a full glass of water or juice, and then sip it every hour or even less so that you have sipped the entire dose over about 10 or 12 hours. That should knock it out in about 24 hours. Or keep it up until the flu is gone. It never lasts more than 48 hours that way. To knock it out in 24 to 48 hours it takes constant attention. Even 1/2 hour basis is better. Just keep sipping it. A single large dose will stay good for at least 24 hours.

Cystic Fibrosis

What it the protocol for treating Cystic Fibrosis?

Q: I have a question about Cystic Fibrosis. Could you provide more details about treating this debilitating disease. Could you outline a treatment plan?

A: Essentially it is the same protocol. Start at two drops. Keep increasing the number of drops, and if you are not getting well, you are not taking enough. Just work at it. Reach 15 drops three times a day, and take that for a couple of weeks.

Diabetes

How do I know when MMS is the correct 28% solution?

Q: I am up to 17 drops three times a day and am using lime juice to activate it and adding have a glass of water after the three minutes. I can see the change in color of the liquid and the smell as well. However, I am not sure that the MMS is 28% because the liquid that comes out of the green bottle is very clear. I have even put some of on my skin but it did not burn me. The only time the MMS burnt, is when I put it on some fungal spots on my skin. So far, I have not noticed anything different happening with my body but did have a bit of nausea a couple of times. I am a diabetic and am hoping that this product can help.

A: If it turns yellow and its smells, then than is good. When you take MMS, you will feel a little nausea, diarrhea or vomiting; those are good reactions. It says that the MMS and

154

your body are working together, anyways try to increase the dose.

Does MMS cure diabetes?

Q: What about diabetes, does MMS cure diabetes?

A: People do not like me to use the word cure as it upsets some people to even have the concept that something can be cured so I will not say it very often. A group of researchers in Canada have stated that all persons with diabetes have an inflamed pancreas. Many doctors have said that, so it's really nothing new. What is new is MMS. The Chlorine Dioxide created by the MMS overcomes the inflammation of the pancreas and guess what, the symptoms of the diabetes.

Would MMS help me treat type 1 diabetes?

Q: I was just curious if you heard of anyone is healed of type 1 diabetes with the use of MMS or if anyone with Type 1 diabetes has had problems with MMS. Any information would help because I am very interested in it. Even if it does not heal my diabetes, it would be great to be healthier!

A: I have some success stories with all different type of diabetes, I think you should start taking MMS.

Does MMS work with diabetes or complications from diabetes?

Q: Does MMS work with diabetes or complications from diabetes? I have someone who takes insulin shots twice daily, and is on numerous other medications his kidneys are also at 30% and has neuropathy and is blind in his right eye.

A: Yes MMS works really well on people with diabetes. I know of a lot of people who are off their insulin, I also known of people who have gotten their sight back.

Is it possible to get infection at 15 drops of MMS treatment?

Q: I have been taking the drops for the last couple of months, I have a lot of health issues, diabetes, blood pressure and kidneys and prostate, the worse is exhaustion most of the time. I got to 15 drops and 10 drops within 2 to 4 hrs, I had to cut down, it was very hard getting out of bed in the morning. I am taking 15 drops for couple of weeks. The most interesting, had two prostate infections while at 15 drops, I had to resort to the Beck devise to clear the infection, is it possible to get infection at 15 drops? What do you think of all this?

A: First of all you must increase the drops 1 by 1 each day not all at once, when you start feeling bad you have to cut down the drops and when you are feeling better you must increase the drops. When you get up to 15 drops only take it for 1 week and stay at 6 drops once a day.

What effect does that have on my taking MMS just before bed time?

Q: I have Type ll diabetes and my doctor wants me to take insulin at night before bedtime. Is there a problem?

A: Just take your insulin four hours after taking MMS and you should be fine.

How much MMS should I use to treat my diabetes? Will it get me off my insulin?

Q: Is Diabetes treatable with MMS? Will it help me get off my insulin? How much MMS would I have to use?

A: We have known people who had diabetes and where on insulin and when I say where is because they do not use insulin anymore and they also tell us that they feel much better. I think he should do the standard protocol.

My husband has Diabetes, should he stop taking his insulin when he starts taking MMS?

Q: My husband has Diabetes, should he stop taking his insulin when he starts taking MMS?

A: He does not have to stop taking his insulin until he feels good enough that he does not need it anymore have him take the MMS and wait 3 to 4 hours to take the insulin, remember to start at 1 drop and 5 drops of citric acid and increase it by 1 or 2 drops per day till you get up to 15 drops.

I am wondering whether the mechanism on diabetes is microbe or metal related?

Q: I am wondering what the mechanism might be on diabetes? Would it mean diabetes might be microbe related in some cases? Or, metal related?

A: Generally, what is involved with the diabetes is the pancreas being inflamed; MMS gets the inflammation down, thus the pancreas starts working again. However, it is not a solution for everybody, and only half of the people taking MMS have been helped. If the inflammation goes down the problem might be microbe related.

Dialysis

Can a person with 2 organ transplants and on dialysis take MMS?

Q: I am inquiring for one of our customers: Her question: Her son has had 2 organ transplants in the past few years. One was and kidney, the other a pancreas. He has other heart issues due to the transplants and dialysis. She wants to know if taking the MMS would be harmful to him or in your opinion, would it be ok for him to take it.

A: MMS would help. The reason I believe this is that in many different autoimmune diseases, the MMS stopped the disease. This might stump you as it seem that increasing the power of the immune system would just give it that much more power to attack the body, but that does not happen. The reason being, again in my opinion is that all disorders of the body is caused by microorganisms that are in some way growing in the body. MMS kills all such microorganisms. So far no one has indicated a problem with using MMS with transplants. However, I would go very slowly just to be cautious and safe. Start out at 1/2 drop MMS dose. Make a one drop dose and pour out 1/2 of it. Take a 1/2 dose every day for a weeks or so.

Will MMS be harmful if a person has had a transplant or is having dialysis?

Q: I am inquiring for one of our customers: Her question: Her son has had 2 organ transplants in the past few years. One was and kidney, the other a pancreas. He has other heart issues due to the transplants and dialysis. She wants to know if taking the MMS would be harmful to him or in your opinion, would it be ok for him to take it? Thank you for your help.

A: In my opinion the MMS would help. The reason I believe this is that in many different autoimmune diseases, the MMS stopped the disease. This might stump you as it seem that increasing the power of the immune system would just give it that much more power to attack the body, but that does not happen. The reason being, again in my opinion is that all disorders of the body is caused by microorganisms that are in some way growing in the body. MMS kills all such microorganisms. So far no one has indicated a problem with using MMS with transplants. However, I would go very slowly just to be cautious and safe. Start out at 1/2 drop MMS dose. Make a one drop dose and pour out 1/2 of it. Take a 1/2 dose every day for a weeks or so.

Diet

Can you tell me if it's safe to take the MMS and the Indian herb together?

Q: Can you tell me if it's safe to take the MMS and the Indian herb together?

A: Separate them by about 2 hours when taking them.

Can I eat or drink water after using the MMS?

Q: Are we directly allowed to eat or drink after using the MMS? Or do we have to wait an hour before eating any type of food or drinking normal bottled water?

A: You can wait an hour to drink or eat, but that all depends on you. Of course you can drink bottled water, just make sure that what you decide to eat or drink has no added Vitamin C, and if it does, just wait 1 hour.

Digestive System

Can you comment on the enema protocol?

Q: Hello, within your web site, one article mentioned greater effectiveness was achieved using an ENEMA rather than ORAL. Can you comment on this protocol?

A: Enema protocol: Use the basic protocol, that is starting with 1 drop and increasing eventually to 15 drops. Mix up a drink (a dose whatever number of drops it is you are going to use)and put it aside. Clean your colon out a bit with two or three plain water enemas or add a bit of Aloe Vera juice or 1 level teaspoon of salt to the clean out liquid. Then put in the dose of MMS which should be in about 1/2 glass of water (four ounces). If possible keep the MMS dose inside. The colon will absorb it into the walls. Do this once or twice or up to 4 or 5 times a day. Increase in the number of drops of MMS.

Do we need to flush the body of toxins before taking MMS?

Q: On the issue of constipation, this seems also to indicate the need to flush the body of toxins that have bound up the digestive tract. For me its accompanied by severe gas and liver sluggishness sympomology and I have heard this from others.

A: Yes, I would suggest for most anyone having trouble with the bowels to get them cleaned out. My suggestion is the senna herb. This herb causes the bowels to exercise. This exercise is so violent that it makes the bowels sore like muscles that have been exercised to the extreme. The crust and junk that forms inside the bowels are broken loose more quickly than with most colonics. The junk is expelled. It's more natural than colonics. The MMS is then likely to do a better job.

You can send off for senna leafs, but it is simpler to go to WalMart and buy a box of sennosides. They are made from the senna leafs. Buy the maximum strength. Use as many as it takes to get cleaned out.

Do you think it would be OK to do 33 drops of MMS twice a day to rid Lyme Disease?

Q: I suffer from Lyme disease and parasites. Do you think it would be OK to do 33 drops of MMS twice a day to rid my problem?

A: You could take 15 drops 4 times a day, however a better choice would be to do enemas, because the colon dumps the MMS into the plasma of the blood making it go deeper into the body to do enemas you should use 24 to 30 ounce of water and then use about the same dose as you would use by mouth and implanted in the colon that is put it in the colon and leave it if possible start at 4 or 5 drops of activated MMS and continue increasing by mouth. Do it 2 times a day.

Since I am pregnant, Is the six drop dosage powerful enough to kill worms?

Q: I am breastfeeding my one-year-old child. A friend of my husband told us about your product MMS and wrote to you about whether it is safe to take while breastfeeding. You said it was safe, but to limit it to the 6 drop dosage. I believe I can feel parasites / worms moving around inside of me and have seen my waste moving around in the toilet. I think my two daughters may have parasites / worms too. On the bottle of MMS, it says that the 15 drop dosage should be used to kill parasites / worms. My questions are:

1. Is the six drop dosage powerful enough to kill the worms or should I be doing something else? Should I take a drug to kill the worms and then take your product? Also, is the child and baby dosages strong enough to kill the worms in the kids?

2. Can I take the 6 drop dosage and give the baby dosage to my one-year-old (breastfeeding) daughter at the same time?

3. My 5 year old daughter, husband, and I have been taking MMS for 4 days. We are up to 4 drops once a day, taking one extra drop each day. How many times a day should we be taking MMS?

162

A: Go for 15 to kill the worms, But go slowly working up to that does one drop at a time. You can take the MMS from one to three times a day. Look at how you feel and how much you think you can take without making yourself too nauseous. It is good for babies, but if the baby becomes nauseous you might have to use a bottle for a few days, not likely, but maybe. If the 3 drops for 25 pounds of body weight does not do it, use more.

Can MMS help me with gut parasites?

Q: I have been suffering for years with gut parasites, giardia was found in my stool some years ago. Antibiotics have proved ineffective but, I have reduced the infection down greatly with herbal methods. The reason I am writing to you because I am undecided as to the dose I should start off with. In your book you state that one should always start with one drop and build up except in the case of a parasitic problem in which case start at 15 drops. Also, what is the procedure, if nausea comes on too strong or vomiting takes place, as to the second dose of the day? Do I reduce back to one drop and work back up, or just say halve the dose? Finally, because gut parasites are not in the blood, can the immune system aided by the MMS still seek them out?

A: Always start off with 1 drop of MMS 2 or 3 times a day. Increase 1 drop per day until you get to 15 drops 2 or 3 times a day. When you start feeling sick (nausea, vomiting, headache or diarrhea), just lower the dose to the point where you are not feeling bad, once you overcome those symptoms start increasing the dose. What MMS finds it will kill it.

Will **MMS** help me with my digestive problems?

Q: I had digestive problems (from gallbladder removal) and stones still in my liver. I also have atrophied adrenal glands and hypothyroidism from being on too high a dose of hydro cortisone since childhood. Now the dose is affecting my health, but I get withdrawal symptoms and go into crisis when I attempt to reduce. It has been mentioned that your product can strengthen my immune system and help rebuild my adrenal glands. is this true? Also, I have a very sensitive body due to my congenital adrenal insufficiency which can cause adrenal crisis, dehydration and death if not monitored correctly. Will taking your product send the body into intense healing crisis? Is it worth taking to rebuild adrenal cortex tissue? Have you had any suggestion with it this area?

A: I have no experience in this area. However, the MMS has been applied to hundreds of areas where I have no experience. I believe it would help. If you take it start with very little dose say ½ drop or ¼ drop. Use one drop to mix the dose with then pour out one half and add a little more water and drink. In a few hours try a slight larger dose. Work at it. It has a better chance than anything else. Stones in the liver can be dissolved with olive oil. For a normal person it works good with ½ glass of olive oil blended with ½ glass of lemon juice maybe twice in a day. Immediately lay on your right side for an hour. I have done if for myself a few times and have had quite a few others do it.

Has anyone gotten back to you on success stories about using **MMS** for Ulcerative Colitis or Crohns disease?

Q: I received my MMS in the mail yesterday and was wondering if anyone has gotten back to you about success stories about using MMS for Ulcerative Colitis or Crohns disease.

A: We have had a few reports of success with those diseases; use the standard protocol.

If someone has hemorrhoids or Crohns disease, would the mix of MMS and citric acid make this worse?

Q: If someone has hemorrhoids or Crohns disease, would the mix of MMS and citric acid make this worse?

A: Citric acid should not make the hemorrhoids or crohns disease any worse.

Has anyone gotten back to you about success stories on using MMS for Ulcerative Colitis or Crohns disease?

Q: I received my MMS in the mail yesterday and was wondering if anyone has gotten back to you about success stories about using MMS for Ulcerative Colitis or Crohns disease.

A: We have had a few reports of success with those diseases; use the standard protocol.

What would be the best and most effective protocol to use MMS for stomach ulcers?

Q: What would be the best and most effective protocol to use MMS for stomach ulcers?

A: Take MMS slowly start at 1 drop, do not use vinegar use citric acid, lime or lemon for activation. To dilute the solution use some juice but do not use juices that have added vitamin C. Increase the dose by one or two drops a day. If you experience nausea, diarrhea, or vomiting just decrease the dose by one or two drops. Once the symptoms are gone increase the dose again.

Will MMS assist with diabetes, arthritis, stroke victims and constipation?

Q: Will MMS assist with diabetes, arthritis, stroke victims and constipation?

A: Yes it will help all of those conditions.

Is it normal to have cramps and diarrhea after taking MMS?

Q: Is it customary to have cramps and diarrhea? I am taking 15 drops twice a day.

A: Yes it is normal to have cramps and diarrhea that means that your body is getting rid of all the toxins in your body, keep on taking MMS just decrease the dose to the point where you are not feeling sick. Then increase it again.

Will MMS work for autoimmune conditions that affect the function of the colon?

Q: My girlfriend has an autoimmune condition affecting the function of the colon. Are there any reports so far on the effects of MMS on autoimmune conditions?

A: Autoimmune problems have been overcome using MMS by improving the function of the immune system.

Would MMS react with Infliximab?

Q: My son who is 18 years old has Crohns disease, he has been on an immune suppressant Infliximab, and I wanted to know if he takes MMS would this react with the Infliximab.

A: MMS dos not react to any drug as long as you separate them by 2 hrs or more. Just start with small dose 1 drop or less and see if there is a problem.

Is there another activator other than citric acid that can be used to activate the MMS?

Q: I was wondering if there is a activator that's more easy for me to tolerate. It seems the vinegar/lemon lime juices all irritate my stomach. I have had trouble with ulcers and have found a magnesium mix of magnesium and citric acid also irritates me. Are there any alternatives that will activate the MMS? I thought maybe if I drank a few glasses of water before I used the mix it might help.

A: Those are the only activators proven effective so far. It's because they are acidic. Be sure your stomach is full when you take the MMS. A full stomach will help prevent the irritation. However, the MMS should very soon overcome the ulcers, so take small does for a while until the ulcers are gone.

Does MMS help peptic or gastric ulcers? Does it grow hair?

Q: I am a pretty healthy person except for some stomach problems and was wondering if you have a list for potential cures. Does MMS work on helping hair grow? Does this help with peptic or gastric ulcers?

A: MMS helps get rid of ulcers just keep increasing the dose. I have not done any test on hair but I have heard of people telling me their hair has growing back.

What can I do if I am having trouble going up to 15 drops a day?

Q: My wife and I were extremely excited to try your MMS. As instructed, we started off with 2 drops twice a day, adding another drop every day. I ended up getting to 12 drops a day. That day I got a little diarrhea, so I cut back to 11 drops a day. I did this for another couple of days and then went up to 12 drops a day. I did 12 drops a day for 2 days and then the diarrhea hit me big time. I would like to finish my initial treatment and get up to 15 drops, twice a day for 2 week, to make sure I have removed all the toxins in my body, but I am afraid my body would end up rejecting the treatment. Any ideas on what I might do?

A: It is normal to have diarrhea just lower the dose to the point where you are not feeling bad when you start feeling better increase the drop if it happened again you have to do the same thing lower the dose then increase, diarrhea means that your body is eliminating something bad from your body. Do not stop taking MMS continue taking it eventually you will get to the 15 drops. The microorganism load is generally very large. It may take a while. The body does not reject MMS, at lease no cases of that so far. For taste please see that section of this book.

Is it normal that I get nauseous after taking MMS? Will it cure me from Hepatitis C?

Q: I experienced extreme nausea which built up gradually, then bowel cramps starting in upper bowels and working its way down, and finally diarrhea. I wanted to see if I could cure the hep-c so it would not show up on conventional blood tests any longer. After all, it is a virus.

A: It is normal to get nausea, diarrhea or vomiting, those are good indicators that mean that MMS is working and is eliminating bad stuff from your body. Now the thing is that you do not want to make yourself that sick, so lower the dose you are taking to the point where you are not feeling sick. You are doing a great job, just lower the dose and you will be fine. Once the sickness stops just increase the dosage slowly again. Keep it up until you are free of Hep C. That may take several months, or less.

Does not feeling any nausea mean that MMS is not working?

Q: Never felt any nausea. Is it a good/bad sign? Does it not mean that MMS is unable to find any bad stuff in the body to oxidize?

A: It is normal for someone to not experience any nausea, vomiting or diarrhea. Just wait until you get to 15 drops 3 times a day. And you are right, there was very little to oxidize but that does not mean that some very dangerous pathogens were not killed.

What's the most recommendable dosage to start off with if I am not sure whether I still have gut parasites?

Q: The reason I am writing to you because I am undecided as to the dose I should start off with, I have ordered some MMS from Canada. You state that one should always start with one drop and build up except in the case of a parasitic problem in which case start at 15 drops. I do not know for sure if there is any giardia left, only a very strong suspicion as any test for it is very inconclusive. So not sure what to do, my instinct is to start at 15. I have always had some nausea since this problem started, which is why I believe I still have parasites.

Also, what is the procedure, if nausea comes on too strong or vomiting takes place, as to the second dose of the day? Do I reduce back to one drop and work back up, or just say halve the dose? Finally, because gut parasites are not in the blood, can the immune system aided by the MMS still seek them out?

A: Always start off with 1 drop of MMS 2 or 3 times a day, increase 1 drop per day until you get to 15 drops 2 or 3 times a day. When you start feeling sick (nausea, vomiting, headache or diarrhea), just lower the dose to the point where you are not feeling bad. Once you overcome the sickness, start increasing the dose once again. The immune system seems to be able to find the parasites with MMS present. I would reserve the 15 drops dose to begin with only if I was sure the parasites were present.

Will the MMS be able to find and kill parasites and toxins located within the gut?

Q: So you are saying that the MMS is perfectly capable of finding parasites and toxins that are within the gut itself?

A: If it exists, MMS will kill it.

Will MMS work on Hep C, Thrombocytopenia, Leukytosis, Crohn's Disease, Ankylosing Spondolitis, Osteopenia, Chronic severe Insomnia and Inflammatory, Rheumatoid, Degenerative and Osteo Arthritis?

Q: I have Hep C, Thrombocytopenia, Leukytosis, Crohn's Disease, Ankylosing Spondolitis, Osteopenia, Chronic severe Insomnia and Inflammatory, Rheumatoid, Degenerative and Osteo Arthritis. Will I be able to use this product safely?

A: Yes you will be able to use MMS safely if you follow the protocol starting off with 1/2 drop of MMS. Follow the standard protocol, but be very slow to go to each new increase of MMS. Remember, when you feel sick, just lower the dose a few drops. MMS will help you with many of your diseases.

How long can someone stay on 15 drops of MMS once a day?

Q: How do I know how long to take MMS after I reach 15 drops once a day? I have had parasites due to a bird mite infestation and want to strengthen my immune system. I also have high cholesterol so I want to take it for that. I am up to 9 drops and am experiencing diarrhea and stomach cramping. I know it says this is a normal reaction, but should I continue increasing the dosage?

A: When you experience diarrhea, nausea or vomiting just lower the dose to 1 or 2 drops. When this stops, starts increasing the dose again, until you get past that sickness.

Stay 1 week at 15 drops (if you are well you can take it 2 or 3 times a day.) After that week stay at the maintenance dose of 4 or 6 drops a day for older people and 4 to 6 drops twice a week for younger people.

Will MMS help ease peptic or gastric ulcers?

Q: I am a pretty healthy person except for some stomach problems (possible ulcers.) Does MMS help with peptic or gastric ulcers?

A: MMS helps get rid of peptic and gastric ulcers. Follow the MMS protocol and just keep increasing the dose.

Will MMS react with the inflixmab, an immune suppressant?

Q: My 18 years old son has crohns disease. He has been on inflixmab, an immune suppressant. If he takes MMS would this react with the inflixmab?

A: MMS does not react to any drug as long as MMS and the drug are separated by 2 or more hours. Just start with a small dose of 1 drop or less and see if there are any problems.

DMSO

What may be a simple protocol for using both MMS and DMSO together?

Q: I have the following simple questions:
1-On page 6 of Chapter 3, third paragraph last line; you wrote that "The solution then continues to generate chlorine dioxide for the next 12 hours in the body" However, on your CD conversation (MMS: What you Need To Know) you mentioned that "there is no build up of chlorine dioxide in the body because it only last for two hours". Please clarify??

2- Also, during your CD conversation, you mentioned that Chlorine Dioxide may be taken with DMSO. For educational purposes, from your experience, what may be a simple protocol for using both factors together?? Also, what are possibly 2 or 3 good source of quality DMSO?

A: Each single piece of chlorine dioxide only lasts for 2 hours. The entire MMS dose continues to generate pieces of chlorine dioxide for about 12 hours, that is less and less over a period of 12 hours. When taking MMS and DMSO I always mixed the MMS and DMSO together just before swallowing. I generally used one tablespoon of DMSO with various amounts of MMS. However, I started in the beginning to use several drops, then more drops, then more drops until I was taking 2 tablespoon fulls each dose. I would recommend 1 tablespoon full each dose for several weeks to evaluate how the DMSO is helping.

What form/concentrate of DMSO would be used (or how) with a stroke?

Q: What form/concentrate of DMSO would be used (or how) with a stroke?

A: Use 90% DMSO or 99.9% DMSO.

Do you think that the MMS will eventually kill giant tape worms? Should I have it injected into my spine?

Q: I had some tests done, and I have three different giant tape worms. They are not in my intestine they are in my spine. I have been on the MMS now for one month. Do you think that the MMS will eventually kill them? Should I have it injected into my spine?

A: Yours is a special case so let me suggest a special technique use MMS mixed with DMSO, DMSO has been use by 100 of thousands of people no record of anybody being hurt and it penetrates everywhere in the body and it will carry the MMS with it. My suggestion is you start with a few drops of MMS and increase the drops slowly until you are around 10 continue to increase the MMS but begin taking DMSO first in 2 or 3 drops then go to 10 drops 15 drops, then to a tea spoon then to 2 tea spoons each time about 20 to 40 minutes after you take the MMS finally take up to 2 table spoons but do not start off that way and keep that up for as long as it takes to kill those worms off. These is just a suggestion I am not a Dr. DMSO is a material much like kerosine but penetrates everything.

What is DMSO and where can I purchase it?

Q: My mother has had a couple of mild strokes and I heard that DMSO will help her. What is DMSO and where can I purchase it?

A: You can buy DMSO from a natural health food store. You can go to any search web page and type in DMSO.

Does MMS need to be taken with DMSO?

Q: I have a son who is undergoing some unorthodox treatment for cancer which treatment uses DMSO? I noticed on the bottle that it mentions to not take the miracle mineral supplement until 72hrs after taking DMSO. Should MMS be taken with DMSO?

A: There is no liability in taking the DMSO and the MMS at the same time. In fact, they aid one another to some extent. However, if you do take them at the same time. Start out will small amounts and work up to larger doses. Then also take MMS at a separate time as well, like 4 hours later. Protocol is always started at two drops or less. We are talking about cancer and about 4 months. So I would take MMS every 4 hours or so. Starting at about 1 drop. If that went OK, go to 2 drops on the next 4 hours. If that goes OK go to the 3 drops. Somewhere along the line nausea will set in. When that happens, reduce the drops, but do not stop. As long as nausea occurs, reduce the drops. Wait for a time or two and increase the drops by 1. Just keep that up. The underlying principle is always, if you are not getting well, you are not taking enough.

Can I take DMSO with MMS?

Q: I have a Veterinarian client who is now taking MMS, thanks to you! However, he's been on DMSO for years. He asked me to question you as to why one cannot take DMSO with MMS? Your answer would be appreciated.

A: There is no problem with DMSO and MMS. That's old data. I have proven beyond a doubt that there is no problem.

Is there a reaction between DMSO and MMS that you know of?

Q: I received the MMS, and used 2 drops yesterday afternoon. I had used DMSO gel on my knees to help with some stiffness (had knee replacements about 6 months ago) yesterday morning. About 12 hours later I experienced severe itching under the skin around my knees and some slight nausea earlier.

I checked the instructions from GL more closely and noticed that they suggested waiting 72 hours after using DMSO before using MMS, something I had not seen in your instructions. Is there a reaction between DMSO and MMS that you know of? The itching is subsiding this morning, so it's nothing serious but I thought you would want to know about it.

A: There is no problem with taking DMSO and MMS. That problem has been settled. No doubt the MMS was attacking some anaerobic growth. It is a good sign. Keep at it.

Can I use MMS on a radiation burn?

Q: Have you ever used MMS on a radiation burn? What do you suggest here?

A: I would use a drop of DMSO mixed with a drop of MMS that has been previously activated; put it on in a tiny spot, wait a few hours to see what happens in that spot, then the next time, cover a bigger area.

Where can I obtain and how can I use DMSO in combination with MMS to treat breast cancer?

Q: I am using this MMS on my 27-year old who has stage IV breast cancer. I listened to the CD that came with my order. In the CD you mention that you use DMSO with MMS. I would like to know where to obtain this DMSO and how to use it. I would like my daughter to use MMS with DMSO to beat her cancer.

A: Lots of health food stores have begun to carry DMSO again.

What would be a good ratio to convert DMSO to liquid?

Q: Your friend in Alberta included a note not to use DMSO with the basic protocol. Yet another contact says to use it in the same ratio as the mineral. You have mentioned using it in book two, so I am curious about its use. If DMSO comes as a powder, what would be a good ratio to convert it to liquid? Please let me know where the DMSO stands.

A: DMSO is sold as a liquid, and it cannot be made into a powder. Try making kerosine into a powder. There is no liability in using DMSO and MMS together. Normally, I would add the lime or lemon juice to the drops of MMS and then wait the three minutes and then add an equal amount of DMSO. Use that directly on the outside of the skin to kill cancers and other things. Add water or juice to that to drink. DMSO stops the action of MMS slowly after a period, so if you are not getting results, use them separately.

Edema

Will the highest dose harm me if I continue with it since my edema and lumps are not completely gone?

Q: I have been on the higher doses for two weeks which is what you suggested and want to know if you think it will harm me to continue as the edema is not all gone and the lumps are not completely gone?

A: It will not harm you to continue the higher dose until you are well.

Can MMS help severe Dental Infections in both Teeth and Jaw Bones?

Q: I have been diagnosed with Hypothyroidism resulting from severe dental infections in my teeth and jaw bones for many years. I have had 8 teeth removed and the infections scrapped out. But I am told I should have all my teeth removed and have my entire jawbone scarped out to clear all of the infection. I have been told my thyroid is destroyed and my immune system weak. I am very swollen with edema as a result of my body's attempt to deal with all the remaining infections. Will the MMS help this situation?

A: The first thing you need to do is overcome the infections in your mouth. Make up a 10 drop MMS solution with 50 drops of citric acid. Wait the 3 minutes and add half a glass of water to that.

Use a soft toothbrush and pour the solution onto it. Brush your teeth and gums 3 or 4 times a day.

See how your gums are doing after a week of doing this. Chances are they will be well in a week.

Finally go to a health food store and buy some iodine solution. Start taking 2 drops and work your way up to 30 drops a day to make sure that your body gets saturated with iodine.

Do not worry about over doing the iodine. Just increase the dosage slowly as you need to have all your body's organs saturated with iodine, before finally starting to slowly come off any medication you may have been on.

Endogenous Retrovirus

Does stabilized oxygen work with MMS? Will this formula help with Endogenous Retroviruses and Lyme Disease?

Q: Is the Stabilized Oxygen OK to use with the vinegar/juice formula? It has deionized water, potassium chlorite and sodium bicarbonate? Will this formula help with Endogenous Retroviruses? Will MMS also help get rid of my Lyme disease?

A: Stabilized oxygen does not work with MMS, it will not create the chlorine dioxide, as far as Lyme disease is concern it should help you, I think that enemas are the most effective way against it. Flush the colon out first with water and aloe vera or a teaspoon or two of baking soda. Then flush out the baking soda. Then implant the MMS just as if it were a dose to be taken by mouth. Keep increasing the drops until you reach at least 16 drops per implant. Leave it in as long as possible. It should all be absorb into the sides of the colon.

Eye and Vision Disorders

Does MMS work with diabetes or complications from diabetes?

Q: Does MMS work with diabetes or complications from diabetes? I have someone who takes insulin shots twice daily, and is on numerous other medications his kidneys are also at 30% and has neuropathy and is blind in his right eye.

A: Yes MMS works really well on people with diabetes. I know of a lot of people who are off their insulin, I also known of people who have gotten their sight back.

What do you know about using MMS topically in eyes?

Q: What do you know about using MMS topically in eyes?

A: Yes you can use it in the eye, I recommend making a 6 drops of MMS and 30 drops of Citric Acid solution, if you use lemon juice filter it trough a Coffee filter, allow the 3 minutes to activate and then add about 1/8 water of glass to that, then use that as drops for the eye and dint leave it in the eye longer from 3 to 5 minutes and then wash it out with purified water or eye wash.

Should I continue using MMS on a 1 year 10 months child with Retinoblastoma if his eyes seem to be heating up?

Q: I am trying MMS on a child of 1 Year 10 months who has Cancer in her eyes (Retinoblastoma). I started giving her two drops, with lemon juice and the three minutes wait. I recently increased to three drops. Then I notice that her eyes heat up very much. Should I continue using it?

A: That is a good indicator, but back off to fewer drops to where it does not hurt. Heating up is just a herxheimer reaction which means a result of a die off so reduce the number of drops until that is not happening.

What are the protocols for treating cataracts and HIV?

Q: I just wanted to know if MMS can be used on one of my patients suffering with cataracts. Also, what is the protocol for HIV if I am also using iv insufflation along with MMS for patients.

A: It is OK for patients with cataracts to take MMS. The Protocol for HIV is the same as given below for standard protocol.

Fibromyalgia

Should I stop taking medication for my fibromyalgia?

Q: I forgot to ask this: I am taking Gabapentin tablets for my fibromyalgia and wondered if I should stop taking them?

A: You do not have to stop taking your medications. Just separate your intake by 3 or 4 hours.

MMS does not interfere. But we do suggest people to separate them. It is your decision to stop taking your medications, for you know when you are ready to stop taking them.

Does the MMS work on Fibromyalgia?

Q: I was just wondering if you knew about the condition FIBROMYALGIA? Could you kindly tell me if you know of the condition and of any positive results using your formula? I am now 51 years old.

A: There have been some people with Fibromyalgia who have reported good results, but they never get back to me, so I do not know if they are fully recovered. You should give it a try and let me know how everything goes.

Fungi

How do I prepare for MMS treatment? Can I take probiotics?

Q: I still have questions about using MMS with Candida. My MD has diagnosed me with systemic candida.

1. I know because of my age (57 years) I need to take care with use of MMS because it will strip out the yeast, revealing the pores and pits in the circulatory system caused by candida. I have been taking vitamin C and Calcium with Magnesium for a month in an attempt to prepare for MMS therapy. Is there anything else I can or should do to prepare?

2. I would like to continue to take the beneficial probiotics that help keep the gut clear of candida. When can I take them after MMS dosage? When can I take the Vitamin C ?

3. I took a one drop dose as an experiment. I had very slight shortness of breath a half hour after taking it. I do not normally have SOB and wonder if that was a problem.

A: Just get on the MMS. The C was a good idea. Take the vitamin C 3 or 4 hours before or after taking the MMS, Beneficial probiotics about 1/2 hour away. The shortness of breath was a good sign. However, keep taking one drop until shortness of breath does not occur. You can take one drop every 3 hours or so, checking for shortness of breath each time. When shortness of breath no longer occurs then go to 2 drops and do the same. Only go to larger doses when there are no herxheimer reactions.

I had some reaction towards MMS, is this normal?

Q: I was having a severe reaction to the MMS (I thought) I started with one drop 2 X a day. I never get sick but a couple of days after starting it I developed a sore throat, fever, coughing, phlegm, pain behind my eyes, exhaustion. But he said it may have been something I picked up and the MMS just enhanced the virus. I am up to only taking 3 drops twice a day. I had no nausea, but today the diarrhea came. I read some people get a little cold and sometimes a sore throat but nothing like this. Just wondered if there had been cases like this and a detox reaction. Also, a friend has been getting conflicting info on whether or not MMS gets rid of Candida. The latest info she found from a distributor said that there is still testing going on with that specific problem and it has not been verified. I appreciate any info or advice.

A: Sorry to hear about your problem, however, it is not something that is unique. Probably 95% of the people who use MMS get diarrhea. In other words that is nothing new. Being cold and having nausea up to the point of throwing up and even projectile throwing up is not new. When your body thinks that the poison in your stomach should not go through the digestive system you will throw up. Sorry about that, but if you would read my book you will find that the way you avoid these unpleasant reactions (which are all good indicators as they tell you something in your body is being killed and the resulting poison from dead pathogens is being expelled) is to go slow. When you notice a little nausea, do not take a larger dose, take a smaller dose. Then adjust your doses two or three times a day so that you do not get nausea or diarrhea. MMS if effective against Candida, however one must use the proper protocol (directions).

What do you recommend for people with fungus/yeast type gut conditions or female yeast infections?

184

Q: MMS is doing a killer job with pathogens that are more acid based than the human body. It would seem to have no effect on conditions that create an alkaline ph. Many people with fungus/yeast type gut conditions - or as in female yeast infections - would seem to be over looked by MMS? What do you recommend?

A: So far, I have received a number of email and phone calls saying MMS has overcome fungus and yeast type gut conditions and yeast infections in females. For the female, I would prepare a 6 drop standard dose as if one were going to drink it with a full glass of water. Then use that for the female cleanse.

You see, just because an alkaline condition is created, that does not mean that the skin of the pathogens is not still acidic. You cannot measure the pH condition of the pathogen unless you have a laboratory and equipment and knowledge for the purpose.

What amounts would you recommend for a group of forty people who are fasting with me over the weekend and want to try MMS as well?

Q: I have a group of forty people who are fasting with me over the weekend and I wanted to try the MMS with their fast. I usually give them a drink of apple cider vinegar every three hours during the fast as well as many mineral supplement and a lemon drink with spray dried lemon, aloe vera, enzymes, probiotic and rice bran. What amounts would you recommend. Most of the people are motivated to lose weight as well. I was thinking a drop every three hours in their apple cider vinegar drink. I think you mentioned that it is ok to mix in more than a teaspoon of vinegar. We put two teaspoons of apple cider vinegar in a glass of oxygenated water. We could also add one drop of MMS every three hours in the drink. If they experience vomiting or pain then we could then not give more.

A: Yes, you can do about everything you suggest here. However, I might suggest as time goes by to switch over to citric acid as vinegar which is a fermented product feeds candida. In Tijuana at a large clinic they found that using vinegar with MMS worked for about two weeks, and then the people got worse, those that had candida, this is. I have thousands using citric acid and it seems to work very well. When they switched over to citric they all got better.

What's the protocol for treating chronic sinus problems and for yeast overgrowth? How can I treat my dog that has Cushing's disease?

Q: I am interested in taking MMS for chronic sinus problems and for yeast overgrowth. I would also like to give it to my dog that has Cushing's disease. I am going to order MMS, but would like to know a recommended dosage for my 8 lb. Maltese.

A: Do the standard protocol. For animals, use 3 drops for every 25 pounds of body weight.

Do you think MMS might effect or cure rather extreme toenail fungus?

186

Q: What would you recommend as a maximum dose to work up to? Do you think it might also effect or cure rather extreme toenail fungus?

A: The maximum dose is 15 drops 3 times a day; it will work inside and out.

Is MMS ever used topically for toenails or dry spots or melanoma spots?

Q: Is it ever used topically for toenails or dry spots or melanoma spots?

A: Yes it has been used topically, what you can do is put it directly on your toe, what I suggest is putting it directly on the toe with the fungus mix for example 6 drops of MMS with 30 of citric acid and a table spoon of water and splash it on your toes you can leave it there over night or a few hours and just rinse it. For the melanoma spots take a 2 ounce bottle and mix 20 drop of MMS and 100 drops of citric acid solution wait 3 minutes and fill the rest of the 2 ounce bottle with water, spray it on your melanoma 2 or 3 times a day and keep taking MMS by mouth.

Can MMS help me with Hepatitis C, Lupus and fungus nail problems?

Q: I have Hepatitis C and slightly elevated liver enzymes. I have Lupus and some fungus nail problems. I am a kidney dialysis patient. Can MMS help me with your formula?

A: All lupus cases so far have indicated that are gone, the viral count should reduce dramatically I do not know how long it will take, some people take longer than others. Anywhere to 2 weeks to 2 months take MMS so you can get ride off Hepatitis C.

Does the MMS work in conjunction with probiotics and maintenance of good flora and good bacteria?

Q: Your MMS sure helped my really swollen throat situation. I stopped taking for a while, I felt I needed a break. I have a couple questions: Does the MMS work in conjunction with probiotics and maintenance of good flora and good bacteria? For candida or I suppose any condition, it would be fair to say that since the efficacy is good for 3-4 hours, it is best to take at least 2X a day if not three, correct? Is it ok to take the MMS when one is eating as well as on an empty stomach?

A: It is best to take it on an empty stomach but if you prefer to eat just wait an hour then take MMS, also you could do the maintenance dose which is also on my web page. Remember for candidas do not take MMS with vinegar because vinegar feeds candida, use citric acid, lime or lemon.

The question is if MMS can affect the overabundance of Candida throughout the body?

Q: The question is if MMS can affect the overabundance of Candida throughout the body?

A: I am not sure, I totally understand everything you said but many people have used MMS for over coming Candida problems I do not know what that means that the Candida is all gone that is hard to prove, many parts of the body require an acidic condition in order for the body to live all though thousand of people subscribe to the ideas that the body must be alkaline in order to prevent disease, that is barley theory has been proven in cadavers, a dead person is always alkaline, the body requires a lot of acidic condition from one way to the other.

If I got sick by taking 5 drops of MMS should I increase this dose or lower it?

Q: I have suffered with chronic fungal infections and bacterial infections and have mercury poising for ten years. I have tried MMS but it made me sick at 2 drops should I take more or less?

A: Stay at 2 drops for a week, then start increasing the drops 1 a day so you can pass the 2 drops you have to go all the way up to 15 drops, but on your way to the 15 drops if you get sick again lower the dosage, remember that when you get nauseous or diarrhea is a good indicator which means you are eliminating some bad stuff from you system. Also it's OK to take MMS if you have mercury, do not worry about that it will get rid of it. But remember your goal is to go up to 15 drops 2 or 3 times a day for a week. Then after a week go to the maintenance dose.

Is it possible that herpes outbreaks will eventually stop with the 5-6 drops a day regimen over the course of years?

Q: I have herpes and I am having a lot of difficulty sustaining the regular 10-15 drops twice a day due to nausea and fatigue.

In fact, I can barely make the 6 drop once a day thing and I have had a bad flu despite this regimen. And now the flu after 3 weeks is subsiding the herpes is making a comeback. I took 10 drops with vinegar last night and two hours later the herpes was active, so at 6 am the next morning I took 10 drops again, and within an hour I was vomiting and with severe stomach cramps. Is it still effective to take the drops at a minimum and although have outbreaks, is it possible that they will eventually stop with the 5-6 drops a day regimen over the course of years perhaps? Why, after taking it regularly would this flu be so intense and last this long?

A: First of all, do not take MMS with vinegar, vinegar feeds Candida so stop using it and use citric acid, lime or lemon. Generally herpes is one of the harder things to handle but they can be handled, just keep increasing the doses to at least 15 drops 3 times a day for a week or 2 then check and see if not keep it up. It will eventually get it.

Do you have any protocol for external application of toe nail fungus?

Q: I am up to 4 drops and will move up to 8 tonight. Do you have any protocol for external application of toe nail fungus?

A: Yes, for toe nail fungus just apply directly to the affected area for example you can put some on before you go to bed leave it on overnight and remove in the morning by taking a shower.

Does MMS kill or eliminate Candida and parasites?

Q: Does MMS kill or eliminate Candida? Does MMS kill or eliminate parasites?

A: Yes MMS will help with Candida and parasites, just take MMS with citric acid, lime or lemon.

Is it OK to use lime juice instead of vinegar?

Q: I have worked my way up to 8 drops of MMS to 16 drops of vinegar now three times and at this point the smell makes me nauseous and when I cut back a drop or two I still have the same feeling to the point that I must go off it for a while until I can smell it without feeling sick. I was wondering if it would be OK to add lime juice instead.

A: I would prefer if you take it with citric acid, lime or lemon, I do not suggest you take it with vinegar, because vinegar feeds Candida. To omit the taste or smell I suggest you drink it with juice that has no added vitamin C.

Would MMS help combat a bacterial infection in the sinuses and Candida?

Q: I was about to start the MMS protocol for my Candida problem, when I came down with a bacterial infection in my left maxillary sinus. Would MMS help combat a bacterial infection in the sinuses as well?

A: Yes it will help you. Just use the standard protocol.

Is MMS a good substitute for antibiotics?

Q: We have put our daughter on this product just recently, (she is 16), she was required to have long term antibiotics that we did not want her to take, is this product a good substitute for the antibiotics?

A: I do not know if she can use it as a substitute, but I do know that MMS will help her. Now if she has toe fungus what I suggest is putting it directly on the toe with the fungus mix for example 6 drops of MMS with 30 of citric acid and a table spoon of water and splash it on your toes you can leave it there over night or a few hours and just rinse it.

What is artificial vitamin C?

Q: What is artificial vitamin C?

A: Vitamin C is used as a preservative. That means it preserves. In order to produce chlorine dioxide, the sodium chlorite must deteriorate. Vitamin C preserves it from deteriorating. Natural C that is a part of the fruit does not seem to do that. Lemons contain citric acid. It's the citric acid that we need. Citrus is not the same thing. Vinegar is a fermented product. Fermented products feed candida. All the patients using vinegar with their MMS began to get worse until we changed to Lemon. I hope that answers the questions.

Is it safe for a person to receive intravenous treatment by mixing MMS with vinegar?

Q: I just spoke with my friend who treats his cancer with MMS intravenously now for a few days and asked him for more details. He said, his doctor believes, that glucose might nourish the cancer. So he used NaCl solution without glucose. But instead of mixing it just with the MMS drops and wait for one hour, his doctor recommends 22 drops of the MMS with 2 tablespoonful of ordinary vinegar and wait for three minutes and then mix that into 500ml IV solution. My friend took this IV mixture several times now, but felt very weak and cold after it (shivering/ague). (He is a very thin man who mainly eats raw fruit). I just told him, that the other organic ingredients in the vinegar might bring some unwanted material into the blood and thus cause immune system reaction or maybe even allergic reaction. (I personally would not recommend that vinegar procedure at all, but I am no medical doctor.) But his doctor seems to see it as a kind of additional stimulation therapy.

What do you think? Have you any comments or hints?

A: That was about the craziest thing I have heard so far. That could have killed him. Well, anyway now we know that one can live through 22 drops and vinegar. So far as I know you friend is the first man in the world to ever take that much solution activated into his veins. Amazing. As far as I know, I was the first man to use activated MMS in the veins and I did that starting 3 weeks ago with 7 infusions working up to 4 drops and 26 drops of citric acid, waiting 3 minutes and mixing it into the saline IV solution.

Do you see? Hundreds of thousands of infusions have been done but no one ever mixed the vinegar or other acids with the sodium chlorite. That's new. The cold chills I had with only 4 drops. Do you see, I and he is the only ones so far to run chlorine dioxide through the veins and he 6 times ahead of me. Wow! Well now we know.

Now I think that will be the most effective of all against cancer, but my suggestion is that they drop far back to say 8 drops, with 20 drops of 10% citric acid solution, wait 3 minutes mix it into a 250 ml solution and then do the infusion. (500 ml has been several doctors as too much liquid. It is thought that it could cause water in the lungs). If he does not have the chills then work slowly up to 22 drops. But anytime he gets the chills, use less drops. The chills and being weak are an indication that the body is destroying something but do not destroy it too fast.

Some people have mentioned that 22 drops in a 250 ml bottle might make the solution too strong. But one simply uses the same amount of time as with the 500 ml and the blood dilutes the solution as it hits the vein. It results in the same thing with less water.

I am glad that you have informed me so far. It might be best that he use the citric as at least one clinic has found that vinegar tends to feed Candida.

Can both precancerous spots (keratosis) and the Herpes Virus be treated successfully with MMS?

Q: As far as skin cancer goes - would precancerous spots (keratosis) respond to MMS, and would it need to be applied topically to work or is ingesting it enough?

With herpes virus, I was wondering if MMS actually eliminates the virus from the body (versus just eliminating or controlling an active outbreak)? Do you know of any cases where a person got a herpes blood test after treating with MMS and the test was negative?

A: For skin cancer. Mix one drop of MMS with 5 drops of lemon or citric acid solution and wait 3 minutes. Now, take 3 drops of that solution and add to 3 drops of DMSO and mix it together. Put it on the cancer immediately. If you need more than 3 drops, use four or five or more and always use the same number of DMSO drops. If it is cancer, it will begin to burn right away and the burning should not last long. Maybe 3 to 5 minutes. Once the burning has stopped, cover the area with Vaseline, and cover that with a bandage of some kind. The cancer should come out within a day or two. Do not pull it out. It might come out with the bandage. Make sure you get enough drops on it to kill it the first try so when it starts to burn you could add a drop or two of MMS. Most skin cancers are cured simply by taking MMS by mouth, but not always. If it burns but does not go away, it might be some form of fungus.

Generally herpes is one of the hardest things to handle but it can be handled. Just keep increasing the doses to at least 15 drops 3 times a day for a week or two, then check and verify your progress. If not, keep it up. It will eventually get it. We have heard of people feeling much better with MMS, but we do not have the before or after blood tests to make sure they are completely cured, if you get any verification let me know.

Does MMS do a good job in eliminating Candida?

Q: Does MMS do a good job in eliminating Candida?

A: I have had some reports of people recovering from

Candida. They do not get back to me, so I do not know if they are fully recovered. Why do not you give it a try and let me know how everything goes.

Can I also use MMS externally if I have Candida and MRSA infection in my skin?

Q: I have suffered from a parasitic infection since 2002. I have got Candida really bad now from all the antibiotics and the MRSA infection in my skin is really bad on my scalp, abdomen, privates and all over my rear. So I have a few questions:

Is it better to use MMS with fresh squeezed lemon juice or the citric acid?

Can I use it externally, if so mixed in olive oil or a natural creme?

A: It is basically the same. It is up to you with what ever you prefer to take it with. Yes, it can be used externally. Get a small 2 ounce spray bottle and mix 20 drops of MMS with 100 drops of citric acid solution or lemon juice, wait 3 minutes, add the mix to the 2 ounce bottle and fill the rest of the bottle with water. Spray it on your affected area 2 or 3 times a day and let it dry. If it stings when you spray it on, reduce the strength of the solution by diluting with 50 percent water; also keep taking MMS orally. There is a solution suggested there that has worked for many people. In your case I would suggest following the suggested procedure as many people with this kind of skin infection have been helped. It's rare, but when a person has a skin infection that simply will not go away and it seems to get worse, it's not what they think. The fungus protocol works almost every time.

Can cider vinegar be used as an activator of MMS?

Q: Can apple cider vinegar be used as an activator of MMS?

A: I would recommend you use citric acid, lime or lemon juice as an activator of MMS since vinegar feeds Candida.

Gout

Is there any information available on uric acid & gout?

Q: Do you have any information on uric acid & gout?

A: I do not have any information except that people tell me that they are feeling much better from gout after they have taken MMS.

Would MMS work on gout?

Q: You ever had gout? When you are oxidizing too much stuff in your body and the your body has no way of metabolizing the uric acid by-product - it crystallizes out into little needles - and you get gout, So carrying on would have been very uncertain indeed, the most likely outcome an increase in pain.

A: Other people with gout have noticed an improvement when taking MMS; you just have to take small amounts. MMS makes your body more able to get rid of those poisons that you are talking about.

Gum Disease

How do I use MMS to cure gum disease?

Q: For gum disease, how exactly do I use it when I have brushed my teeth? Do I flush with MMS? How much is needed and for how many seconds do I keep it in my mouth for the cleaning?

A: Use 10 drops of MMS and 50 drops of citric acid, take a gentle brush and soak it into the MMS solution. Brush your teeth and gums 3 or 4 times a day for the first week or two. In 3 or 4 weeks, you will see a big difference. You may also use the MMS solution as a mouth wash. Once your gums are hard and not bleeding, and there is no soreness, you can revert to brushing only 3 or 4 times week.

Hair

Can I use MMS together with a hair treatment for hair growth?

Q: I am looking at a hair program called 'Regenix'. As a part of their treatment they use chlorine dioxide in an aqueous solution as a part of their treatment topically for the cleansing of your scalp. Do you know if I would be able to use your product in the same fashion? This is an excerpt from their patent, "Chlorine dioxide with a range from 100 to 1000 ppm, more preferably 100 to 500 ppm, even more preferably about 250 to 500 ppm." If the chlorine dioxide source contains higher levels, it can be diluted using an appropriate solvent. For example, the chlorine dioxide can simply be diluted in water.

Alternatively, the chlorine dioxide can be diluted in a commonly available hair care base. The diluent, however, should not be so strongly buffered that it becomes difficult to render the chlorine dioxide sufficiently acidic upon application of the acidic solution to break down the chlorine dioxide.

The preferred pH range for the acidic solution is from about 3.8 to 4.2. Citric acid and/or ascorbic acid are the preferred acidic species used to provide the desired pH, but practically any biologically compatible acid can be used, so long as it can achieve the desired pH."

A: MMS is used at concentrates of 10 ppm and less. They use a hell of an amount of ClO2 at 500 ppm except one thing. ClO2 does not work at the pH levels they suggest very well. 3.8 is definitely too low. Maybe that's why it does not do a lot of damage. A few people have mentioned that their hair is growing back, but not many.

What is the best way to control sores on ones head?

Q: What is the best way to control sores on ones head?

A: Mix a 6 drops drink as if you were going to take it. Be sure to activate it with the 30 drops of citric acid. Wait three minutes and then add 1/4 to 1/2 glass of water. Soak or comb this drink into your hair. You can rinse your hair in 10 minutes to prevent the hair from bleaching out to blond. It will not bleach white, but it will bleach blond after about 2 to 3 weeks if you treat it every day. However, once or twice a week will kill the sores on your head and if rinsed out in 10 minutes to 1/2 hour it will not bleach your hair. If the sores are really bad you may need to do it every day for a week or even two weeks, but several treatments will usually do the job.

Has anyone mentioned that they saw hair re growth after using this MMS?

Q: Has anyone mentioned that they saw hair re growth after using this MMS?

A: Yes I have a success story of a man losing his hair and he started taking MMS and in a few weeks he noticed his hair growing back.

Does MMS help with hair growth and peptic or gastric ulcers?

Q: I am a pretty healthy person except for some stomach problems and was wondering if you have a list for potential cures. Does MMS work on helping hair grow? Does this help with peptic or gastric ulcers?

A: MMS helps get rid of ulcers just keep increasing the dose. I have not done any test on hair but I have heard of people telling me their hair has growing back.

Can MMS restore healthy hair growth?

Q: Does MMS work to restore healthy hair growth?

A: I have not done any tests on hair but some people have reported to me that their hair is growing back after following the MMS protocol.

Heart Conditions

Does MMS help Heart Attacks?

Q: Does MMS help Heart Attacks?

A: A number of people have reported that their heart condition was improved since beginning to take MMS. One man who was having small heart attacks every day was no more having heart attacks after taking the MMS for three days. Several persons who began having heart palpitations after taking MMS reported later that they felt that their heart was in better condition. The palpitations could be caused by killing bacteria growth on the heart valve.

Would MMS increase the rate at which carbs are being burned and thus cause heart palpitations?

Q: I have been taking MMS for about 4 days and having a reaction that is really bothering me - heart palpitations. Someone from the Lyme forum said that MMS, being a strong oxidizer, increases the rate at which cabs are burned and that if you already burn carbs readily this would add to that effect is this true?

A: MMS is a weak oxidizer and cannot oxides carbs. If the heart palpitations continue you should take small dose of MMS very small several times a day and try and stay below the level of causing heart palpitations but do not stop taking it.

Will MMS help my Idiopathic Dilated Cardiomyopathy (IDC)?

Q: Will MMS help my medical condition which is idiopathic dilated cardiomyopathy?

A: We have not known of someone with your condition, but trust me if this cures Cancer and a lot of other disease it will help you too, why do not use start using it at 1 drop per day and keep increasing as the days pass by go up to 15 drops for a week, then go back to 6 drops which is the maintenance dose and increase again if you wish to. Remember that by increasing MMS you might feel, dizzy, nauseous or even have diarrhea so if that happens just lower the dose and then when you feel better increase the dosage.

I am taking 1/2 aspro to thin the blood as I had a stint in my Carotid artery in my neck. Would taking MMS affect that in way would it or cause the blood to clot?

Q: I am taking 1/2 aspro to thin the blood as I had a stint in my Carotid artery in my neck. Would taking MMS affect that in way would it or cause the blood to clot?

A: As of this day no one has reported bad results with stints, just separate aspro and MMS by 3 to 4 hours.

Will it be ok for my husband to take MMS if he has stints in his heart and is a diabetic?

Q: Will it be all right for my husband to begin the MMS process? He has 5 stints in his heart and is diabetic. He does take a small amount of insulin once a day. Is it ok form him to do this?

A: I have not had any bad report with regard to stints. When your husband takes his insulin and MMS, separate them by two to three hours. Start the doses low and gradually increase them.

Will MMS help me get rid of cancer of the pericardia and palpitation?

Q: I have cancer of the Pericardia, the lining around the heart and lung cancer and now bone cancer. I am convinced that your mixture will work. Will I have enough time to get rid of the cancer? Main question is I also have super ventricular tachycardia and I take Inderal 10mg 2 times a day for palpitation, will MMS cause palpitation?

A: I cannot tell you for sure how long it will take to get rid of the cancer everyone responds differently. If you take it slowly you will be fine just do not rush it, I have heard that some people do cause palpation's, but that's because they do not follow instructions, so just take 1 drop once or twice and increase 1 drop a day. If you feel bad or weak just stay at 1 drop until you can handle that 1 drop.

If palpitation occurs, take less MMS. For instance take 1/2 drop of MMS by dumping out 1/2 of the solution before you drink it. Take less, but do not stop. You will eventually overcome the palpitations.

Can my husband use MMS if he has five stints in his heart arteries?

Q: My husband has had operations twice to put stints in his heart arteries. He now has 5 stints. We would like to know if this product can still be used even though he has the stints. He is also diabetic and takes a small amount of insulin once a day.

A: Your husband can take MMS juts give him small amounts, if he is taking medication just wait 2 to 3 hours.

When MMS turns into table salt is it not harmful for high blood pressure?

Q: After a period of 12 hours, the MMS turns to table salt. Is not this harmful for high blood pressure or heart problems?

A: MMS turns to approx. 10 ml of table salt that is about 1/2 the size of a pin head you could probably not taste it in a half glass of water, and besides all that the idea that salt causes high blood pressure is just a fable of modern medicine.

Would MMS help with stroke caused be atrial fibrillation?

Q: Can you tell me if MMS would help with stroke caused be atrial fib. I have some damage from the stroke, a slight weakness on the left side and a dropping of my right eyelid. Would it help get oxygen to the damaged parts of the brain and would it in any way help with the atrial fib?

A: It's best to use DMSO to recover from a stroke. Use quite a bit, maybe 2 or 3 large tablespoons twice a day or even more. MMS may help.

How long can someone stay on 15 drops of MMS once a day?

Q: How do I know how long to take MMS after I reach 15 drops once a day? I have had parasites due to a bird mite infestation and want to strengthen my immune system. I also have high cholesterol so I want to take it for that. I am up to 9 drops and am experiencing diarrhea and stomach cramping. I know it says this is a normal reaction, but should I continue increasing the dosage?

A: When you experience diarrhea, nausea or vomiting just lower the dose to 1 or 2 drops. When this stops, starts increasing the dose again, until you get past that sickness.

Stay 1 week at 15 drops (if you are well you can take it 2 or 3 times a day.) After that week stay at the maintenance dose of 4 or 6 drops a day for older people and 4 to 6 drops twice a week for younger people.

Is the fact that MMS turns to sodium chloride harmful in any way?

Q: It has been stated that after a period of 12 hours, the MMS turns to table salt. Is this harmful for high blood pressure or heart problems?

A: MMS turns to approximately 10 ml of sodium chloride table salt, which is only about half the size of a match head. You could probably not taste it in a half glass of water and besides the idea that salt causes high blood pressure is just a fable of modern medicine.

Heavy Metal Poisoning

Does MMS flush out bad and good metals and minerals in the body?

Q: Does the MMS help in flushing these and other metals from the body? Given that metals are not living organisms does the MMS process work? And if it does work, what is to prevent the MMS from removing necessary minerals, such as calcium, magnesium, in addition to or instead of the dangerous ones?

A: The dangerous metals are dangerous because they do electrical damage to the body and they are at a pH level that the MMS recognizes. It oxidizes the heavy metals and they then wash out. That is assumed as the tests for heavy metals come up negative after taking MMS when it was positive before taking MMS. The necessary minerals do not do the same damage, and do not have the same electrical characteristics or the lowered pH levels. Do you see? There is a big difference between heavy metals and other metals and chlorine dioxide recognizes that difference. I, on the other hand, do not guarantee anything. That is what we assume as many thousands of people have gotten better. There are very few guarantees in life, but we all try. No one has complained of noticing a deficiency of the good minerals after taking MMS in the past 10 years.

Will MMS help rid my body of the toxins and heavy metals that are in my system from taking psychiatric drugs?

Q: Will MMS help rid my body of the toxins and heavy metals that are in my system from taking psychiatric drugs?

A: Normally it helps with psychiatric drugs, sometimes a little bit, and sometimes a lot, and sometimes not at all. About heavy metals: We tested people for heavy metals then gave them the MMS for a couple of weeks, and then tested them again and they tested free of the heavy metals. However, the test that we used was the roots of hairs pulled from the head. This is supposed to be a good test, but others have said that it is not a good test. Not all of the problems from drugs can be attributed to heavy metals, but we have had good results from the use of MMS with drugs. Just start at 1 drop or 1/2 drop and work one's way up by increasing 1 drop each day. Have them follow the standard protocol.

If I got sick by taking 5 drops of MMS should I increase this dose or lower it?

Q: I have suffered with chronic fungal infections and bacterial infections and have mercury poising for ten years. I have tried MMS but it made me sick at 2 drops should I take more or less?

A: Stay at 2 drops for a week, then start increasing the drops 1 a day so you can pass the 2 drops you have to go all the way up to 15 drops, but on your way to the 15 drops if you get sick again lower the dosage, remember that when you get nauseous or diarrhea is a good indicator which means you are eliminating some bad stuff from you system. Also it's OK to take MMS if you have mercury, do not worry about that it will get rid of it. But remember your goal is to go up to 15 drops 2 or 3 times a day for a week. Then after a week go to the maintenance dose.

Can your product help me with heavy metal poisoning?

Q: I was told that I have heavy metal poison (mercury, cadmium, lead) in my system. I also, lately started having problems with memory and concentration and so on. I would like to know if your product is good for detox for heavy metals and can it help me with the mental issues I am having?

A: The MMS works good for heavy metal removal and all kinds of detoxification.

Hepatitis

If MMS is seeking and destroying acids, would it not destroy and render inactive the stomach acids?

Q: If MMS is seeking and destroying acids, would it not destroy and render inactive the stomach acids?

The reason I ask this is after the large doses it seemed like my digestion was not working and when I ate I had a lot of burping. I am very sensitive to this, due to the sluggish liver from HCV.

A: MMS is not seeking and destroying acids. It cannot destroy acids. It is seeking and destroying pathogens. MMS does not destroy stomach acids. Thousands of people have taken MMS and there is no report of stomach acid being affected. The burping is probably coming from anaerobic bacteria being destroyed.

Is there anything one should be aware of before starting MMS treatment?

Q: I have a friend that has hepatitis C. Is there anything that he should be aware of before using this solution? Perhaps you may have a recommendation for how others have had success with this condition.

A: Most of the people with Hep C who have taken the solution have felt better and some have check free of the virus. Those who did not check free simply did not bother to get a test. Use the standard protocol.

Will MMS work on Hep C if I am not taking other medication for it?

Q: I have hepatitis C, I am wondering if this will work for Hep C. I did not want to take Interferon and Ribivarin! I can handle nausea and diarrhea for the good of my body, but those drugs kill everything in sight. That's why I like what I am reading. It only goes after diseased stuff. Why are medical doctors so ignorant?

A: Medicine is not calculated to cure people. Only to keep them sick so they will continue paying. So far, all the Hep C cases that used MMS have been cured but one. And that one may be cured and not know it. Just follow the standard protocol.

Will I need to stop taking the MMS after I have the inoculations against hepatitis and tetanus for traveling to Vietnam?

Q: I am really impressed. People around me have gone down heavily with flu for several days and bedridden as well. I had one bad night and after increasing the dose to 15 drops it killed the virus. Will I need to stop taking the MMS after I have the inoculations against hepatitis and tetanus for traveling to Vietnam?

A: Keep up the good work. I think you should not get a vaccination and you should take MMS wile traveling to Vietnam MMS will also protect you from diseases.

Can MMS help me with Hepatitis C, Lupus and fungus nail problems?

Q: I have Hepatitis C and slightly elevated liver enzymes. I have Lupus and some fungus nail problems. I am a kidney dialysis patient. Can MMS help me with your formula?

A: All lupus cases so far have indicated that are gone, the viral count should reduce dramatically I do not know how long will it take, some people take longer than others. Anywhere to 2 weeks to 2 months take MMS so you can get ride off Hepatitis C.

Should I go up to 15 drops if 10 made me feel ill?

Q: I am currently up to 8 drops twice a day, I got up to 10, but started feeling really ill, so I lowered it. I found out I had hepatitis-c 5 years ago and when I found MMS, I decided it was time to kill it once and for all. I started in early January and now as it gets a little tougher I am wondering if I should go to 15 drops, twice a day, and then 3 times a day for a week or more?

A: It all depends on you and how far you want to go, you could take 15 drops 3 times a day that is ok. Just take it for 1 week and then lower the amount to the maintenance dose which is 6 drops and 35 drops of citric acid you can do the standard protocol which is on my web page. When you get sick do like you are doing it lower the drops.

What is the protocol for Hepatitis C?

Q: I have been dealing with Hep C most of my life, I am 60 and still in great shape but have an appointment next month in Vancouver, BC to be analyzed by the Transplant Team regarding a new Liver. I have ordered some solution and would like to get some info regarding how to go about dosing myself for Hep removal and Liver cleansing.

A: You should just do the protocol. That is start off at 2 drops and increase drops each day. At some point along the way go to two doses a day. Say around 8 drops increase to 2 doses a day. Then when you get to 12 drops or so increase to 3 times a day and go on up to 15 drops 3 times a day. Just work up to it. When you can take 15 drops three times a day, it should be gone and your liver should be healthy.

Have you any advice or knowledge of hepatitis C sufferers recovering and totally clearing the virus?

Q: I have hepatitis C and wonder if the liver will have problems processing this. Have you any advice or knowledge of hepatitis C sufferers recovering and totally clearing the virus?

A: I know of people with Hepatitis C and they say they feel much better after taking MMS. The liver should have no problems processing the supplement.

What would be a good protocol for Hepatitis C?

Q: What would be a good protocol for Hepatitis C and/or HIV or AIDS as I have family members with these diseases?

A: This protocol will work with many diseases including, patients with Hepatitis C, HIV, or AIDS, colds, flu, pneumonia. They should be evaluated for the present level of sickness. If they are feeling not badly sick (not really nauseous) they should be started off beginning with the 6 and 6 protocol. That is they should take 6 drops and if there is no noticeable nausea, they should have the second six drop dose in one hour. The reason for this is that there seems to be a benefit in shocking the system. This dose is calculated to be a small shock to the system, but it has been very successful over a period of time and several hepatitis C patients have reported good results from the shock theory. The best time of the day for this treatment would be during the morning hours before noon. The treatment should be at least one hour after eating breakfast or anytime one hour after eating.

Note: All mention of drops of MMS in this paper assumes that 5 drops of citric acid solution will be added for each drop of MMS, one waits 3 minutes, and then adds ½ glass of either water or juice.

In the event that the patient does OK on the 6 and 6 drop dose suggested above, on the second day the treatment should go to 7 and 7. This means 7 drops, wait one hour and then do a second 7 drops. The third day the treatment can progress to 8 and 8. This continues until the patient is taking 15 and 15. Anytime there is any slight sign of nausea, the doses for the next day are reduced by 1 to 4 drops depending upon the severity of the nausea.

Anytime the patient feels nausea he is give a full glass of water to drink. If the nausea does not stop immediately, the patient should have a second glass with a level teaspoon of vitamin C added or baking soda. To determine if one should use vitamin C or baking soda at this point evaluate the condition of the patient. If he feels acid in his stomach, use baking soda, and if he feels no acid, use vitamin C.

If the patient appears to be somewhat sick he may not be able to handle the shock. In this case he should be started out at one drop in the morning and one drop in the evening. In the unlikely even that one drops makes him nauseous revert to ½ drop. Each day the dose in the morning and the evening is increased by one drop. When nausea occurs, reduce the number of drops for the next dose. Follow the instructions given above for nausea.

In either case given above the goal is to reach 15 drops 3 times a day for at least one week before testing to determine if the Hepatitis C, HIV, or AIDS is gone. In the event that the disease is not gone the treatment at 15 drops at least 2 times a day should continue for at least 3 months with tests every 2 weeks to determine if the Hepatitis is gone or tests can be conducted less often if money or facilities are not available.

Children can be handled in the same manner except using smaller doses. The maximum dose (equivalent to 15 drops for an adult) is 3 drops for each 25 pounds of body weight and one drop for a new baby. Start children off with one drop and increase from there.

Maintenance doses should continue at 6 drops a day for people over 50 and 6 drops twice a week for younger people.

Is it normal that I get nauseous after taking MMS? Will it cure me from Hepatitis C?

Q: I experienced extreme nausea which built up gradually, then bowel cramps starting in upper bowels and working its way down, and finally diarrhea. I wanted to see if I could cure the hep-c so it would not show up on conventional blood tests any longer. After all, it is a virus.

A: It is normal to get nausea, diarrhea or vomiting, those are good indicators that mean that MMS is working and is eliminating bad stuff from your body. Now the thing is that you do not want to make yourself that sick, so lower the dose you are taking to the point where you are not feeling sick. You are doing a great job, just lower the dose and you will be fine. Once the sickness stops just increase the dosage slowly again. Keep it up until you are free of Hep C. That may take several months, or less.

Can I take your supplement while on Hepatitis C treatment?

Q: I am presently doing the treatment of Hepatitis C which is Interferon and Ribasphere. My question is: Can I take your supplement while on treatment or should I wait until I have completed it? Also by taking your treatment have you had the results of the Virus Hepatitis C being destroyed or going in remission?

A: You can take MMS while being on treatment. Just leave a 3 to 4 hour period apart from the MMS. I have had several people tell me they tested clear of Hep C virus after taking MMS. Unfortunately, I do not have the before and after blood tests for a great many people to make sure Hepatitis C is being destroyed; I only now what people tell me, they claim they feel much better and doing much better.

Is it safe to use MMS if I am also taking immunosuppressant drugs?

Q: I had a successful liver transplant in '05, but have Hep C that is attacking my new liver. I take the immunosuppressant Prograf so I do not reject my new organ. Do you think it's safe for me to use MMS?

A: Yes it is ok to take MMS. Just take it slowly; start at 1/2 drop per day and then gradually increase the dosage. Remember to stay beneath the point where it makes you feel nausea.

Will MMS work on Hep C, Thrombocytopenia, Leukytosis, Crohn's Disease, Ankylosing Spondolitis, Osteopenia, Chronic severe Insomnia and Inflammatory, Rheumatoid, Degenerative and Osteo Arthritis?

215

Q: I have Hep C, Thrombocytopenia, Leukytosis, Crohn's Disease, Ankylosing Spondolitis, Osteopenia, Chronic severe Insomnia and Inflammatory, Rheumatoid, Degenerative and Osteo Arthritis. Will I be able to use this product safely?

A: Yes you will be able to use MMS safely if you follow the protocol starting off with 1/2 drop of MMS. Go to one of my sites listed below and follow the standard protocol, but be very slow to go to each new increase of MMS. Remember, when you feel sick, just lower the dose a few drops. MMS will help you with many of your diseases.

Herpes

What is the best way to control sores on ones head?

Q: What is the best way to control sores on ones head?

A: Mix a 6 drops drink as if you were going to take it. Be sure to activate it with the 30 drops of citric acid. Wait three minutes and then add 1/4 to 1/2 glass of water. Soak or comb this drink into your hair. You can rinse your hair in 10 minutes to prevent the hair from bleaching out to blond. It will not bleach white, but it will bleach blond after about 2 to 3 weeks if you treat it every day. However, once or twice a week will kill the sores on your head and if rinsed out in 10 minutes to 1/2 hour it will not bleach your hair. If the sores are really bad you may need to do it every day for a week or even two weeks, but several treatments will usually do the job.

Can MMS help get herpes out of my body forever?

Q: A few months ago I found out that I have genital herpes. Can MMS help get herpes out of my body forever?

A: Generally herpes is one of the harder things to get rid of but you can get rid of it, just keep increasing the doses to at least 15 drops 3 times a day for 2 weeks.

Can MMS cure Herpes and HIV?

Q: I wanted to know if MMS can cure herpes and HIV?

A: Yes we have had great results with herpes and HIV just use the standard protocol.

How much MMS would someone have to take to get rid of genital herpes?

Q: How much MMS would someone have to take to get rid of genital herpes?

A: Generally herpes is one of the hardest things to handle but they can be handled, just keep increasing the doses to at least 15 drops 3 times a day for a week or 2. It will eventually get rid of it.

Have you had any clinical testing done on someone who has had herpes that has done the 15 drops three times a day for a week?

Q: Have you had any clinical testing done on someone who has had herpes that has done the 15 drops three times a day for a week?

A: I have no before and after test results. People claim they are better but they never get back to me.

I was wondering what success you have had with the Herpes II virus?

Q: I was wondering what success you have had with the herpes II virus?

A: Generally herpes is one of the hardest things to handle, but they can be handled, just keep increasing the doses to at least 15 drops 3 times a day for a week or two. I have received email from people that have taken MMS and said that their herpes has cleared up.

Can MMS be applied directly on cold sores? Can it help with Herpes?

Q: I am on maintenance dose of 6 drops a day. Yesterday I woke up with a large cold sore (herpes) just below my lower lip. My top and bottom lip are swollen on the same side with very tiny herpetic blisters. Can you advise me as to dosage? Should I increase the dose? Can I use the solution directly on the infected area?

A: Generally herpes is one of the harder things to handle but they can be handled, just keep increasing the doses to at least 15 drops 3 times a day for a week or two. You should see an improvement after that. You can also apply the solution directly on the blister once a day but do not leave it on too long apply it for 30 seconds to 1 minute then wash it off.

218

Can both precancerous spots (keratosis) and the Herpes Virus be treated successfully with MMS?

Q: As far as skin cancer goes would precancerous spots (keratosis) respond to MMS, and would it need to be applied topically to work or is ingesting it enough?

With herpes virus, I was wondering if MMS actually eliminates the virus from the body (versus just eliminating or controlling an active outbreak)? Do you know of any cases where a person got a herpes blood test after treating with MMS and the test was negative?

A: For skin cancer. Mix one drop of MMS with 5 drops of lemon or citric acid solution and wait 3 minutes. Now, take 3 drops of that solution and add to 3 drops of DMSO and mix it together. Put it on the cancer immediately. If you need more than 3 drops, use four or five or more and always use the same number of DMSO drops. If it is cancer, it will begin to burn right away and the burning should not last long. Maybe 3 to 5 minutes. Once the burning has stopped, cover the area with Vaseline, and cover that with a bandage of some kind. The cancer should come out within a day or two. Do not pull it out. It might come out with the bandage. Make sure you get enough drops on it to kill it the first try, so when it starts to burn you could add a drop or two of MMS. Most skin cancers, however, are cured simply by taking MMS by mouth, but not always. If it burns but does not go away, it might be some form of fungus.

Generally herpes is one of the hardest things to handle but it can be handled. Just keep increasing the doses to at least 15 drops 3 times a day for a week or two, then check and verify your progress. If not, keep it up. It will eventually get it. We have heard of people feeling much better with MMS, but we do not have the before or after blood tests to make sure they are completely cured, if you get any verification let me know.

By taking this product can one avoid getting shingles?

Q: By taking this product can one avoid getting shingles, because of a person's age and having had chicken pox as a child? Thank You

A: One can avoid getting shingles or chicken pox but if you do contract any of these diseases, what you can do is take MMS by mouth, but also get a small spray 2 ounce bottle mix 20 drops of MMS with 100 drops of citric acid solution, or lemon juice, wait 3 minutes and fill the rest of the 2 ounce bottle with water, spray it on 2 or 3 times a day and keep taking MMS by mouth.

Has MMS been effective treating the Herpes Virus?

Q: I am writing you to ask if you have heard any success stories, or any stories at all relating to the herpes virus?

A: Generally herpes is one of the hardest things to handle but it can be handled. I have people telling me that they do not get outbreaks any more, but they do not tell me if the herpes is gone, since they do not get back to me. What I would do is to continue taking MMS and just keep increasing the doses to at least 15 drops 3 times a day for a week or two; then check and see if any progress has occurred. If not, keep it up. It will eventually get to it.

What is the MMS dosage for Herpes?

Q: I am on a maintenance dose of MMS of 6 drops a day. Yesterday I woke up with a large cold sore (herpes) just below my lower lip. My top and bottom lip are swollen on the same side with very tiny herpetic blisters. Can you advise me as to dosage? Should I increase the dose? Can I use the solution directly on the infected area?

A: Generally herpes is one of the hardest conditions to treat. But it can be controlled by increasing the dose to at least 15 drops 3 times a day for a week or two.

You should see an improvement after that. You can also apply the solution directly on the blister once a day but do not leave it on for too long.

Apply MMS as a topical application for 30 seconds to 1 minute then wash it off.

HIV

I have 2 orphans that are HIV positive, please let me know how to use MMS with them?

Q: I am a missionary in Mozambique caring for 40 orphans. 2 are HIV positive and dear to me. Please tell me more about how to use this medicine with them. One is a girl 6 years and the other a boy 9 years. I have also suffered too much with malaria last year and would like to take it for that. The directions for usage do not seem real clear to me. 2 drops each hour until all the 2 drops add up to 15? I am confused. I am also hopeful.

A: Well, yes, with HIV or AIDS start with one drop and increase each day one drop until you are at 3 drops for each 25 pounds of body weight. For malaria, you need to shock it. Use 15 drops of MMS and 75 drops of activator. Use lemon juice drops as the activator or vinegar or citric acid activator. Wait 1 or 2 hours and hit it with a second 15 drops dose, same as the first dose. That's all you will need.

How will MMS help me if I am HIV positive?

Q: I am HIV positive and how will MMS help?

A: So far as I know it will go into a person's body and kill the HIV virus. I am sure you do not want it to help for the HIV. If you want to know if others have taken the MMS who had HIV the answer is yes. Many have taken the MMS. If you want to know if it made them feel better. Several mentioned that they feel better. If you want to know if they were cured. I do not know. Most people when they get to feeling better do not go to a doctor to find out. They simply go back to their lives.

How do we go about intravenous MMS for HIV patients?

Q: You mentioned giving intravenous MMS to HIV patients. How do we go about it? How many drops (15?) mixed with sterile water?(No citric acid of course). To what proportions? How frequently? And for children? Do the orally doses work well with HIV patients?

A: Do not use sterile water. Us IV solution either saline or glucose or other sugar solutions sold for that purpose. Normally the glucose works best as the saline sometimes causes a drop in blood pressure. If you use a 500 ML bottle start with one drop. Wait and hour after adding the MMS to allow for activation. Use one drop the first day, two drops the second day. Then increase to 6 or 8 the third day. Then increase by 4 to 8 drops a day until you are doing 22 drops in 500 ML of solution in a 2 to 4 hour drip. Normally you would do it until the person is well. Sometimes it works good with HIV patients orally and sometimes you need to do intravenous.

Is taking MMS IV much more efficient than drinking it? Should I stop taking my medication for HIV?

Q: Please treat me as your son and tell me what best should I do to get rid of this HIV virus. Would you tell me to stop my three drugs medication and when? Is it ok to overlap MMS with current medication? Should I take MMS IV if it's much more efficient than drinking it? Stopping medication is a big decision for me to make as I always felt to rely on them in order to live. Please help me with your experience and testimonials.

A: MMS IV is much more effective than taking by mouth. Stop the drugs immediately. HIV is not dangerous. It does not cause AIDS. What causes AIDS is the drugs that you are taking, each one is extremely poisonous. That causes AIDS. The vomiting was a good sign. It means you body is getting rid of bad stuff. It takes a certain amount of courage to stop the drugs, but you really know that they are bad, and that they will not help you live longer. Just depend on the MMS as it is a thousand times better. Read the MMS data a few times. See the logic. Ask yourself that is not more logical than taking poisons.

I wanted to know if MMS can cure herpes and HIV?

Q: I wanted to know if MMS can cure herpes and HIV?

A: Yes we have had great results with herpes and HIV just use the standard protocol that you can find on my web page under important info.

How much does someone need to take MMS to get rid of HIV?

Q: How much does someone need to take MMS to get rid of HIV?

A: I cannot tell you for sure a lot of people who have HIV they say they feel much better or they are doing better, we do not have the before and after blood test to be necessary to do it. However a lot of people say they are negative for aids after taking MMS for a while. If you get any verification please let us know. Start at 1 drop per day, once or twice a day.

Can MMS cure Herpes and HIV?

Q: I wanted to know if MMS can cure herpes and HIV?

A: Yes we have had great results with herpes and HIV just use the standard protocol.

Should I start off with 15 drops if I want to treat HIV?

Q: I have HIV and I just want to find out should I start off with 15 drops?

A: You should start off at 1 drop per day, then start increasing the dosage.

To get rid of AIDS what would you do?

Q: To get rid of AIDS-what would you do?

A: I would start taking MMS start at 1 drop and increase until you get to the 15 drops 2 or 3 times a day as long as you are not getting sick (diarrhea, nausea), you can continue with the 15 drops for a month then do a check up.

Is it better to take MMS intravenously?

Q: I have read that AIDS was treated directly with shots directly into the bloodstream. Is this the recommended method or should I take the mineral by mouth. Should the doses be stronger than normal?

A: Start taking it by mouth, you can also do it by IV, what IV does it goes directly on to the bloodstream.

How much MMS should a patient take to get rid of HIV?

Q: How much MMS should a patient take to get rid of HIV?

A: We do not have before and after blood test to be sure how much MMS you should take to cure HIV or AIDS. However a lot of people say they are HIV negative after taking MMS for a while. Start with 1 drop of MMS and increase the dosage by one or two per day till you reach 15 drops.

What are the protocols for treating cataracts and HIV?

Q: I just wanted to know if MMS can be used on one of my patients suffering with cataracts. Also, what is the protocol for HIV if I am also using iv insufflation along with MMS for patients.

A: It is OK for patients with cataracts to take MMS. The Protocol for HIV is the same as given below for standard protocol. If the HIV is very resistant, you could go to the cancer protocol.

Can you provide us with the details on the IV protocols for cancer, AIDS and other diseases?

Q: My new digital scale with a 1g accuracy did arrive and herewith the required data:

The MMS contents only of our bottles are 100ml and have a weight of 121 gram, our MMS is within the advised +- 5% range. We hope you find this correct.

Further: I think we had today a nice breakthrough for your MMS in South Africa.

My doctor that has been practicing homeopathy for some 40

years. His practice is called "South Africa". He has +- 80 clients per day and has all the latest equipment for blood analysis. He has too many clients with cancer and would only be too pleased if the MMS can help. He would also keep, of course , record for all applications and will have the correct natural medications for boosting the depleted immune system of the sick.

The doctor is very excited to start and asks for the following detailed info as he also wants to use the MMS for IV :

a) what are the protocols for IV for the different CANCER types and

b) what are the protocols for IV for AIDS

c) what are the protocols for IV available for other applications

He further recommended that we sell the MMS with the note : FORMULA 1 and the citric acid with FORMULA 5 (to give reference to the 1 drop MMS to be used with 5 drops of citric acid as advised by yourself for the normal applications) this might be a possibility He further stated..should this MMS be successful with his clients, then he will introduce my company to all the big homeopathy centers in South Africa .

A: Yes, 121 grams is ok. I really meant .5% but 1% or even 2% is acceptable. The exact figure is 122 grams. I would imagine that your 100 ml bottles are not exact either, depending on exactly how full you fill them. We always fill them to the very top to prevent any gurgling or noise of liquid slashing around when the postal people hear it. That always worries them.

That sounds like a wonderful new break through in South Africa.

The IV protocol: For more the 20 years sodium sulfite has been used as an IV solution for various diseases. It has been fairly successful, but it was never activated with the citric acid. I personally tried the activated MMS. That is 5 drops of citric for each drop of MMS. That activated solution was then put into a 250 ml saline IV solution and administered over a period of 1 hour. I noticed a herxheimer reaction of chills for a couple of hours after using only one drop. The next day still using only one drop there was no herxheimer reaction. So I continued to 2 and three and 4 drops. There was always a herxheimer reaction and then no reaction on the second day.

When using activated MMS using 5 drops of citric acid there is no pain. If a pain develops you are doing something wrong. The citric acid of a few drops is not enough to cause pain. Pain results from inserting the needle incorrectly. It is almost always incorrect when using the back of the hand. The best results is using the blood vessels on the arm. If the needle slides along the blood vessel before penetrating the vessel it will cause pain. Try to get the needle to penetrate the blood vessel at the point where it penetrates the skin. Many times after a few days the vessels will knot up and prevent blood flow even when the needle is correctly inserted. This action is standard and one should learn how to use tiny amounts of Heparin and/or Procaine to keep the vessels from rejecting the MMS.

Others have called to tell me that they have successfully treated many different things with MMS IV. The local clinic has treated cancer by MMS IV. As my book says, my doctor treated 390 patients with AIDS. The protocol for AIDS was always to do 6 drops IV 500 ml solution the first day, 12 drops the second day, and 22 drops the third day and continuing thereafter at 22 drops until well. The 500 ml solution was administered over 4 to 8 hours. The 22 drop IV dose is approximately the dose that was use over a 15 year period. Other than the herxheimer reaction of nausea and diarrhea and chills there has never been any adverse reactions to IV treatments.

The reason we may have been successful in Uganda was the 6, 12, 22 drop dose was what one could consider a shock to the system.

The protocol now in the local clinic and most other places is to use 1 drop of MMS the first day, and go to 2 drops only when there is no herxheimer reaction to the IV dose, but continue up to 22 drops watching for herxheimer reaction and continuing to the next higher drops when there is no reaction from the present amount of drops. The IV treatments have always been more effective than by mouth.

What to watch for: If a patient has a drop in blood pressure we have changed the IV solution to glucose rather than the saline solution. When the blood pressure drops, stop the IV and give the patient some fruit juice. Use glucose the for the next day's IV. Check blood pressure if there seems to be a problem. Normally blood pressure is not checked, except very sick or very bad cancer patients.

About the name: Very few people have worried about the name. In fact I have had only one other person who really was worried that it sounded too much like snake oil. He felt that no one would trust such a name, that people would feel that it was bad. But that did not happen. Hundreds of thousands of people have just swallowed it down without a worry about the name. We are several years down the road with the name MMS and Miracle Mineral Supplement.

You see, what I had in mind was what would be most likely to not worry the pharmaceuticals. Miracle Mineral makes the pharmaceutical companies think it is nothing more than all those other mineral doses out there. It is not even in their minds that such a thing could exist. That keeps us below the radar for another few months. AND in the final analysis MMS is going to prove out to be exactly what the name says, it is truly a Miracle Mineral. So I think the name is OK as is.

Nothing wrong with using Formula 1 and Formula 5 to remind people to use 5 drops. That would be OK if you want.

Your bottles sound OK, but remember, MMS will destroy the rubber bulbs on eye droppers. It takes a while, but several months or a year down the road and you have rubber pieces in the MMS.

What would be a good protocol for HIV?

Q: What would be a good protocol for Hepatitis C and/or HIV or AIDS as I have family members with these diseases?

A: This protocol will work with many diseases including, patients with Hepatitis C, HIV, or AIDS, colds, flu, pneumonia. They should be evaluated for the present level of sicknesses. If they are feeling not badly sick (not really nauseous) they should be started off beginning with the 6 and 6 protocol. That is they should take 6 drops and if there is no noticeable nausea, they should have the second six drop dose in one hour. The reason for this is that there seems to be a benefit in shocking the system. This dose is calculated to be a small shock to the system, but it has been very successful over a period of time and some hepatitis C patients have reported good results from the shock theory. The best time of the day for this treatment would be during the morning hours before noon. The treatment should be at least one hour after eating breakfast or anytime one hour after eating.

Note: All mention of drops of MMS in this paper assumes that 5 drops of citric acid solution will be added for each drop of MMS, one waits 3 minutes, and then adds ½ glass of either water or juice.

In the event that the patient does OK on the 6 and 6 drop dose suggested above, on the second day the treatment should go to 7 and 7. This means 7 drops, wait one hour and then do a second 7 drops. The third day the treatment can progress to 8 and 8. This continues until the patient is taking 15 and 15. Anytime there is any slight sign of nausea, the doses for the next day are reduced by 1 to 4 drops depending upon the severity of the nausea.

Anytime the patient feels nausea he is give a full glass of water to drink. If the nausea does not stop immediately, the patient should have a second glass with a level teaspoon of vitamin C added or baking soda. To determine if one should use vitamin C or baking soda at this point evaluate the condition of the patient. If he feels acid in his stomach, use baking soda, and if he feels no acid, use vitamin C.

If the patient appears to be somewhat sick he may not be able to handle the shock. In this case he should be started out at one drop in the morning and one drop in the evening. In the unlikely even that one drops makes him nauseous revert to ½ drop. Each day the dose in the morning and the evening is increased by one drop. When nausea occurs, reduce the number of drops for the next dose. Follow the instructions given above for nausea.

In either case given above the goal is to reach 15 drops 3 times a day for at least one week before testing to determine if the Hepatitis C, HIV, or AIDS is gone. In the event that the disease is not gone the treatment at 15 drops at least 2 times a day should continue for at least 3 months with tests every 2 weeks to determine if the Hepatitis is gone or tests can be conducted less often if money or facilities are not available.

Children can be handled in the same manner except using smaller doses. The maximum dose (equivalent to 15 drops for an adult) is 3 drops for each 25 pounds of body weight and one drop for a new baby. Start children off with one drop and increase from there.

Maintenance doses should continue at 6 drops a day for people over 50 and 6 drops twice a week for younger people.

What is the best time to take MMS?

Q: Am I right in the belief that this is about the nighttime dose's effect on my body, because apart from once, the nighttime dose, even though it's higher, has caused me no problems. In fact, at my best I have been up to 15 drops of a night for several weeks with no nausea or diarrhea. It's the daytime dose, which has always been lower in order that I can maintain my work, that has been the problem. Could you clarify as I am not sure if I should be doing something differently?

Finally, can I say, as a trained naturopath and accredited psychotherapist, your advice has not only been helping me but has been helping my clients and those that I serve, as I am busy beating the drum of the role and value of MMS in our ever-increasingly toxic environment. So I thank you on behalf of myself and those lives you are touching through me.

A: You asked about daytime doses verse night time doses. At night you body has a chance to work on cleaning out the poisons and repairing the damage done while you sleep, but with the day time dose you are not sleeping, you are working or doing other things. It makes you tired. You are probably tired at night too, but you do not notice it as you are sleeping.

Normally, it does not make a big difference if you take 30 or 45 drops. The reason being is that if one is cleaned out at 30 drops, then an increase is going to make no difference. But if you are noticing a difference between 30 and 45 drops it means you are not all cleaned out. MMS does not cause tiredness. It's the dead bacteria or viruses or other dead microorganisms as

233

they dump poison into the system that causes the tiredness. Anyone who is cleaned out should be able to take at least 50 drops without any reaction of tiredness.

Do you see the principle? MMS does not affect the system when there is nothing to kill or clean out (that is in the quantities of MMS that we take. Anything is poisonous if taken in large enough quantities.) I have taken up to 100 drops in a day with no noticeable effect. Others have written me saying the same thing. No one should try that unless they have tried 30, and 40, and 50, and 60 drops a day first. And there is no reason to do that anyway. The microorganisms are gone at much lower doses.

So the principle is to work up to that level (15 drops 3 times a day should be enough), but work up to that level without causing yourself too much discomfort. If you are getting so tired that it is a discomfort to you reduce the amount of drops to the point where you can tolerate the tiredness. Do not allow yourself to have diarrhea. Do not allow yourself to be nauseous, but increase the drops as fast as you can up to the amount that is indicated about. Some diseases take longer than others to clear out. HIV takes a long time, up to 3 months, and maybe even more. Remember, each person is different and will react to MMS differently. But just follow these principles.

What is the appropriate dosage and duration to control/cure HIV?

Q: Would you please respond with the appropriate dosage and duration to control/cure my HIV?

A: Follow the standard protocol. Also, a number of people are getting good results from enemas using the MMS solution. They clean themselves out and then make a standard dose of MMS and use that dose as an implant in their colon. The next day, they increase it by one drop just like taking it by mouth. When using as an implant in the colon, with a little luck they can leave it in, as the colon absorbs water quickly. Using it this way, I think the solution gets deeper and does more good than by mouth but also take it orally.

Will MMS interact with my HIV medication?

Q: I am HIV + and want to give a story of success soon. I will start the protocol as soon as possible. But I have an important question that I wish you can answer prior to start. I am taking a combination of western medication (one a day) ATRIPLA. 1- Should I stop the medicine while doing the MMS protocol? 2- Can I keep taking my daily medicine when using the MMS? 3- Is there any risks by mixing my medicine and MMS?

A: You do not have to stop taking your medications when taking MMS; as there is no risk and MMS does not interfere with medicine. Just separate them by 3 or 4 hours and you will be fine.

How much MMS is required to eliminate HIV?

Q: How much MMS should a patient take to be clear of HIV?

A: A lot of people say that they are HIV negative after taking MMS for a while.

Start with 1 drop of MMS and increase the dosage by one or two drops per day till you reach 15 drops. It may take up to several months to be HIV negative and clear of AIDS.

Hypothyroidism

Does MMS pull our mercury & lead from the tissues as well as the EDTA & DMSA IV treatments?

Q: In trying to figure out why I get sick so often they have discovered I have a serious hypothyroid & my mercury & lead toxicity is off the charts. The doctor I am going to suggest EDTA & DMSA I.V. treatments. Independently, I have read about cilantro as a miracle to detox. Does MMS pull our mercury & lead from the tissues as well as the EDTA & DMSA IV treatments. Do you know of any toxicity from these IV treatments. Is it over kill to do both IV & MMS?

A: MMS has been known to pull mercury and lead out of the tissues. I would give it a good try first as it is much cheaper and in my opinion usually does a better job.

Can MMS help severe Dental Infections in both Teeth and Jaw Bones?

Q: I have been diagnosed with Hypothyroidism resulting from severe dental infections in my teeth and jaw bones for many years. I have had 8 teeth removed and the infections scrapped out. But I am told I should have all my teeth removed and have my entire jawbone scarped out to clear all of the infection. I have been told my thyroid is destroyed and my immune system weak. I am very swollen with edema as a result of my body's attempt to deal with all the remaining infections. Will the MMS help this situation?

A: The first thing you need to do is overcome the infections in your mouth. Make up a 10 drop MMS solution with 50 drops of citric acid. Wait the 3 minutes and add half a glass of water to that.

Use a soft toothbrush and pour the solution onto it. Brush your teeth and gums 3 or 4 times a day.

See how your gums are doing after a week of doing this. Chances are they will be well in a week. Then follow the standard protocol.

Finally go to a health food store and buy some iodine solution. Start taking 2 drops and work your way up to 30 drops a day to make sure that your body gets saturated with iodine.

Do not worry about over-doing the iodine. Just increase the dosage slowly as you need to have all your body's organs saturated with iodine, before finally starting to slowly come off any medication you may have been on.

Immune System

Is it better to take the MMS on an empty stomach or full stomach for best efficacy?

Q: I am about to start the MMS for a chronic periodontal/immune system dysfunction problem and I have a question. I would like to know, is it better to take the MMS on an empty stomach or full stomach for best efficacy?

A: Less likely to get nausea if you have something in your body, but is really only because MMS is much more effective on an empty stomach, you have to pattern your dose in that respect. You can wait from 1 to 2 to 3 hours that all depends on you.

How can I use MMS? Will it help me cure my Sarcoidosis and Erythema nodosum?

Q: I have received 3 bottles of MMS. Why is there no explanation for me on how to use it? It sounds like to me that one has to use it with citric acid powder or liquid? And how does one do that? Why does one have to mix it with citric acid? Do you have any case stories of anyone cured from a 4 year old Sarcoidosis and Erythema nodosum?

A: Most bottle have instructions on it, however the reason for using citric acid is it reduces the acidic level to the point where the MMS will release the chlorine dioxide and of course the chlorine dioxide is what kills the viruses and other microorganisms. Use 5 drops of citric acid for each drop of MMS wait 3 minutes and then add half a glass of juice do not use orange juice.

Does one have to be on the MMS for a prolonged period of time to get the immune system working at its optimum rate?

Q: I have several clients who have been at 15 drops once a day MMS protocol for a month. Once they are done this protocol, they are still coming down with a flu or cold. I am really surprised that they would even get sick, because I thought the MMS would have boosted their immune system enough to offer them protection. Has this been your experience too?? Does one have to be on the MMS for a prolonged period of time to get the immune system working at its optimum rate?

A: Flues and colds both have a psychological component and a body function normally however no matter the flu or cold is if they continue MMS it will only last 2 or 3 days at worst, when I say body function sometimes the body needs to clean itself out and it uses the flu or cold for that, other times when the body sees a cold germ or a flu germ it will turn on the psychological function for a couple of days but in any case that will only last for a short day and it will be gone.

When would be the best time to start taking MMS if I have Wegener's Granulomatosis?

Q: I have a disease called Wegener's Granulomatosis, an autoimmune disease vacuities condition. I am looking forward to receiving the supplement but am unsure when would be the best time to start taking it. I have my treatment once a month and therefore my immune system is really low for the first 10 days. Do you have any suggestions?

A: So far MMS has cured all of the autoimmune diseases, I would wait until you are a few days away from the treatment that you mentioned and follow the standard protocol.

How long do the contents of a bottle of MMS last after opening it? Will MMS boost the immunity of babies?

Q: Once you open a bottle of MMS - how long do the contents last? 2. Dosage for babies? Are babies considered pretty clean (without Candida, parasites) or are some given MMS to boost immunity? If yes, what's the dosage?

A: Once you open a bottle the solution will last you more than a year. The dose for babies is 3 drops for every 25 pounds or for new born babies 1 drop at most 2 drops. As long as the baby is good and healthy I would not bother given them MMS however if they have allergies problems or any other problems I would recommend you give them 1 drop per day and in that case the maintenance dose would be half a drop per day.

How long can someone stay on 15 drops of MMS once a day?

Q: How do I know how long to take MMS after I reach 15 drops once a day? I have had parasites due to a bird mite infestation and want to strengthen my immune system. I also have high cholesterol so I want to take it for that. I am up to 9 drops and am experiencing diarrhea and stomach cramping. I know it says this is a normal reaction, but should I continue increasing the dosage?

A: When you experience diarrhea, nausea or vomiting just lower the dose to 1 or 2 drops. When this stops, starts increasing the dose again, until you get past that sickness.

Stay 1 week at 15 drops (if you are well you can take it 2 or 3 times a day.) After that week stay at the maintenance dose of 4 or 6 drops a day for older people and 4 to 6 drops twice a week for younger people.

Infection

How do I prepare for MMS treatment? Can I take probiotics?

Q: I still have questions about using MMS with Candida. My MD has diagnosed me with systemic candida.

1. I know because of my age (57 years) I need to take care with use of MMS because it will strip out the yeast, revealing the pores and pits in the circulatory system caused by candida. I have been taking vitamin C and Calcium with Magnesium for a month in an attempt to prepare for MMS therapy. Is there anything else I can or should do to prepare?

2. I would like to continue to take the beneficial probiotics that help keep the gut clear of candida. When can I take them after MMS dosage? When can I take the Vitamin C ?

3. I took a one drop dose as an experiment. I had very slight shortness of breath a half hour after taking it. I do not normally have SOB and wonder if that was a problem.

A: Just get on the MMS. The C was a good idea. But get the MMS. You do not want too long of a runway. Take the vitamin C 3 or 4 hours away from taking the MMS, Beneficial probiotics about 1/2 hour away. The shortness of breath was a good sign. However, keep taking one drop until shortness of breath does not occur. You can take one drop every 3 hours or so, checking for shortness of breath each time. When shortness of breath no longer occurs then go to 2 drops and do the same. Only go to larger doses when there are no herxheimer reactions.

Is MMS hard on the liver and kidneys?

Q: Is it a falls belief that MMS is hard on the liver and kidneys?

A: Yes, it is a false belief; MMS cleans up both the liver and kidneys sometimes right away and some times it might take a month or two.

What do you recommend for people with fungus/yeast type gut conditions or female yeast infections?

Q: MMS is doing a killer job with pathogens that are more acid based than the human body. It would seem to have no effect on conditions that create an alkaline ph. Many people with fungus/yeast type gut conditions - or as in female yeast infections - would seem to be over looked by MMS? What do you recommend?

A: So far, I have received a number of email and phone calls saying MMS has overcome fungus and yeast type gut conditions and yeast infections in females. For the female, I would prepare a 6 drops standard dose as if one were going to drink it with a full glass of water. Then use that for the female cleanse.

You see, just because an alkaline condition is created, that does not mean that the skin of the pathogens is not still acidic. You cannot measure the pH condition of the pathogen unless you have a laboratory and equipment and knowledge for the purpose. Just try it out. Give it a chance to do its work. It does not hurt anyone.

Can MMS take the infection out of a tooth?

Q: Can MMS take the infection out of a tooth? Do I understand correctly that bacteria, parasites and viruses that the MMS kills just oxidize? They leave to residue behind for the body to get rid of?

A: Yes it will clear the infection; in fact I know a lot of people who brush with MMS, just prepare it like a normal drink, like if you were going to drink it and then you brush your teeth. I have a lot of success stories with gums and teeth and you are correct it does leave residue behind for the body to get rid of, but in the case of brushing you teeth the residue is a very small amount which you will wash out when you rinse you mouth.

Does MMS push infections to the surface?

Q: I noticed a capped tooth that used to abscess is kinda sore, as is a place in my mouth where I had a wisdom tooth removed eight years ago. Maybe the MMS is pushing the infection to the surface? Also, a lymph node on the side of my neck is swollen to the size of a quarter. I was not sick that I knew of when I started taking this yesterday. And also I used to have muscle spasms in the arch of my foot and upon my first dose of 3 drops of MMS yesterday I noticed a tingling and crawling sensation in that area.

A: In the process of killing the bacteria, virus, mold, and yeast load things get irritated as the microorganisms die out. Make a dose and use the dose to dip you tooth brush in for brushing your teeth and gums. Do it twice a day for a while. You will see a big change for the better. Looks like you are doing great. Keep it up.

Are you aware of any experience with MMS for inflammation or kidney infections?

Q: Are you aware of any experience with MMS for inflammation or kidney infections?

A: Yes it has helped people that had inflammation and kidney infections,

Any suggestions on how long I should stay off MMS for the effects to wear off?

Q: I was able to rid myself of an infection, however I think I may have over done it a bit. After building up for about 10 days I did a dose of 15 to 25 drop doses three times a day. It's been 4 days since I have taken any at all. I was getting rashes all over and red irritated skin. Also dry and almost burdened knuckles…I took a two drop dose today and within an hour I had skin And gum irritation! And loss sensation in the skin. Any suggestions on how long I should stay off MMS for the body to heal?

A: That's the first time I have heard of anybody taking that much or having any damage I would and I am not sure is damage, wait a month and try 1 drop dose you may have just dislodged something, wait a month and take a drop and if it still happens wait another month, but be sure to keep it up.

But remember start at 1 drop.

Can MMS take the infection out of a tooth?

Q: Can MMS take the infection out of a tooth? Do I understand correctly that bacteria, parasites and viruses that the MMS kills just oxidize? They leave to residue behind for the body to get rid of?

A: Yes it will clear the infection, in fact I know a lot of people who brush their teeth with MMS, and they just prepare it like a normal drink, like if they were going to drink it and then they brush their teeth. I have a lot of success stories with gums and teeth and you are correct it does leave residue behind for the body to get rid of.

Does the MMS have any effect on favorable bacteria in the colon such as acidophilus?

Q: I have a client who has a bladder infection diagnosed by his urologist, for which he is taking penicillin. He has completed two weeks of the indicated four week program. Would it be alright for him to start MMS now or should he wait until he is finished with the penicillin in two weeks? Also, does the MMS have any effect on favorable bacteria in the colon such as acidophilus?

A: MMS will not hurt the penicillin. Bladder infections are a snap for MMS and many treated including cancer. No, the MMS does not affect the acidophilus in the colon or anywhere else in the system.

Would it be wise to use MMS on a 9-month old baby with nose, ear and eye infections?

Q: My granddaughter has a sort of cold, nose, ear and eye infection, she is 9 months old has had this for 4 months since day-care. Would it be wise to try MMS?

A: Start at 1 drop several times and then use two drops. You can give it to the baby 1 or 2 times per day. Remember put 1 drop of MMS and 5 of citric acid, lime or lemon wait 3 minutes and add the water or juice. When a baby gets runny nose and stuffed up and MMS does not seem to do much, you can generally count on the baby being allergic to pasteurized homogenized cows milk. You may have to use something other than cow's milk.

How much stabilized oxygen should I use to treat a jaw infection?

Q: I live in South Africa and want to try this for a severe infection in my jaw (the bone, not the gums). I am trying to avoid surgery as my body is not strong enough to handle surgery at present. I do have stabilized oxygen at home and perhaps I could try it. How much should I use? I see you recommend 120 drops. Is there any reason why you sometimes recommend water instead of the fruit juice? I would prefer to use water as I have allergies to many things including most fruits.

A: The stabilized Oxygen might work. For this purpose, I would use about 40 drops. Add about 40 drops of lemon or lime juice, wait three minutes, then add about 1/2 glass of water (about 200 ml). I know the infection is in the jaw, but dip your tooth brush into the solution and brush your teeth and brush your gums. Take at least 5 minutes. Then swallow the remainder of the solution. Do this 4 or 5 or 6 times a day until the infection is gone. If you have true stabilized oxygen it will smell of chlorine after you add the lemon juice. It should say sodium chlorite on the side. The lemon juice is what makes the difference. It activates the stabilized oxygen.

Kidney

Can a person with 2 organ transplants and on dialysis take MMS?

Q: I am inquiring for one of our customers: Her question: Her son has had 2 organ transplants in the past few years. One was and kidney, the other a pancreas. He has other heart issues due to the transplants and dialysis. She wants to know if taking the MMS would be harmful to him or in your opinion, would it be ok for him to take it.

A: MMS would help. The reason I believe this is that in many different autoimmune diseases, the MMS stopped the disease. This might stump you as it seem that increasing the power of the immune system would just give it that much more power to attack the body, but that does not happen. The reason being, again in my opinion is that all disorders of the body is caused by microorganisms that are in some way growing in the body. MMS kills all such microorganisms. So far no one has indicated a problem with using MMS with transplants. However, I would go very slowly just to be cautious and safe. Start out at 1/2 drop MMS dose. Make a one drop dose and pour out 1/2 of it. Take a 1/2 dose every day for a weeks or so. Do not get upset if you notice a change. It might be a good change, but if it seems like a bad change, stop for a few days, and then try it again.

Is MMS hard on the liver and kidneys?

Q: Is it a falls belief that MMS is hard on the liver and kidneys?

A: Yes, it is a false belief; MMS cleans up both the liver and kidneys sometimes right away and some times it might take a month or two.

Will MMS help me with biliary cirrhosis, melanoma on my leg and other numerous physical injuries?

Q: I have massive health problems–congenitally defective kidneys which over the years have caused biliary cirrhosis of the liver–the later I have had for at least twenty years–ten years ago I almost died from brain cancer-and a melanoma on my leg–a woman from Denmark turned up in my life and saved it– but generally my life has been one long nightmare–besides all the sickness–major physical injuries too numerous to mention-i just wonder what you think–my reactions seem outside anything you talk about.

A: Use lemon or lime juice instead of vinegar. Your reactions seem reasonable considering your condition, you should just continue with the MMS. You might want to read FAQ's on the MMS web site. Do not give up. Others who where having similar problems eventually came through. It may take a while.

What can I do if one drop of MMS causes kidney pain?

Q: I have historical problems with kidneys during detoxification regimes. One drop MMS causes kidney pain. Do you have any suggestions?

A: If 1 drop of MMS gives you kidney pain, then what you should do is take half drop of MMS. The way you mix a ½ drop dose is take a drop of MMS put 5 drops of Activator, wait 3 minutes and add half glass of water, get another glass and pour half of the mix to that glass then add water to one of the glasses until it's half full. That is how you make a half drop.

Do you think your product will help me improve my lungs condition?

Q: I had a kidney removed and lymphatic gland somewhere near my lungs, I am doing fine on wheat grass fruit and veggie diet, traces in my left kidney and lung have remained stable for a few years, do you think your product will help me get rid of it altogether?

A: I do not know if it will get rid of it all together but I think it will help you, give it a try and let me know how everything goes, if you have more questions let me know.

Is it possible to get infection at 15 drops of MMS treatment?

Q: I have been taking the drops for the last couple of months, I have a lot of health issues, diabetes, blood pressure and kidneys and prostate, the worse is exhaustion most of the time. I got to 15 drops and 10 drops within 2 to 4 hrs, I had to cut down, it was very hard getting out of bed in the morning. I am taking 15 drops for couple of weeks. The most interesting, had two prostate infections while at 15 drops, I had to resort to the Beck devise to clear the infection, is it possible to get infection at 15 drops? What do you think of all this?

A: First of all you must increase the drops 1 by 1 each day not all at once, when you start feeling bad you have to cut down the drops and when you are feeling better you must increase the drops. When you get up to 15 drops only take it for 1 week and stay at 6 drops once a day.

Will MMS help me with a break out of pimples I have all over both hands and the insides of my forearms?

Q: I had surgery to fix hernias and when I got out of hospital my hands started itching and breaking out with pimples and it has spread all over both hands and the insides of my forearms. I have tried everything and the doctors do not help. Will this help me? Also during my surgery or after my kidneys shut down, after a strong water pill and walking I was able to urinate normally again, but I feel this could be connected?

A: Take a 12 ounce bottle put 20 drops and 100 drops of citric acid wait 3 minutes add the water and the mixture to the bottle and spray it on the affected area, also you should start taking it by mouth start the standard protocol.

Do you think that MMS will help in dealing with a kidney stone that is stuck in the ureter near the bladder?

Q: Do you think that MMS will help in dealing with a kidney stone that is stuck in the ureter near the bladder?

A: Yes it will help you, start at 1 drop per day 2 or 3 times a day and increase 1drop per day. When you get to 15 drops stay at 15 for 1 week. Then lower the dose to 4 or 6 drops which is the maintenance dose a day for older people and 4 or 6 drops twice a week for younger people.

Are you aware of any experience with MMS for inflammation or kidney infections?

Q: Are you aware of any experience with MMS for inflammation or kidney infections?

A: Yes it has helped people that had inflammation and kidney infections.

Have you ever had any experience with your product and Chronic Kidney Disease?

Q: I was wondering if you ever had any experience with your product and Chronic Kidney Disease.

A: It has been in our experience that people take MMS in a period of a couple of months and there kidney clears up and in some cases the kidney appeared to clear up in weeks. So start at 1 drop per day and increase 1 drop each day go up to 10 or 12 drops, remember if he gets dizzy or nausea or vomiting lower the dosage then increase again once he is passed this. Only go up to 12 drops at most.

Will MMS work if I had a kidney removed?

Q: Recently I had a kidney removed and a lympathic gland somewhere near my lungs, I am doing fine on wheat grass / fruit and vegi diet, traces in my left kidney and lung have remained stable for a few years, do you think your product will help me get rid of it altogether?

A: I do not know if it will get rid of it all together, but I think it will help you.

Will MMS help deal with a kidney stone that is stuck in the ureter near the bladder?

Q: Do you think that MMS will help deal with a kidney stone that is stuck in the ureter near the bladder?

A: Yes it will help you. Start at 1 drop per day 2 or 3 times a day and increase by 1 drop per day. When you get to 15 drops, stay at 15 for 1 week. Then lower the dose to 4 or 6 drops which is the maintenance dose a day for older people and 4 or 6 drops twice a week for younger people.

Liver

Is MMS hard on the liver and kidneys?

Q: Is it a falls belief that MMS is hard on the liver and kidneys?

A: Yes, it is a false belief; MMS cleans up both the liver and kidneys sometimes right away and some times it might take a month or two.

If MMS is seeking and destroying acids, would it not destroy and render inactive the stomach acids?

Q: If MMS is seeking and destroying acids, would it not destroy and render inactive the stomach acids?

The reason I ask this, is, after the large doses, it seemed like my digestion was not working, when I ate, a lot of burping. I am very sensitive to this, due to the sluggish liver from HCV.

A: MMS is not seeking and destroying acids. It cannot destroy acids. It is seeking and destroying pathogens. MMS does not destroy stomach acids. Thousands of people have taken MMS and there is no report of stomach acid being affected. The burping is probably coming from anaerobic bacteria being destroyed.

Is it true that by taking the sodium chlorite causes symptoms of liver congestion, or extreme gas in the intestines?

Q: It has been found in different health oriented yahoo groups that taking the sodium chlorite causes symptoms of liver congestion, or extreme gas in the intestines. In other words a very strong need to detox. Some of us feel it as our liver becoming hard, A symptom saying that the liver is fighting to rid the body of whatever the result of taking MMS produces, dead bacteria or toxins. I think it might be wise if you mention a need for detoxing the liver or bowels as part of treatment with MMS. feel it as our liver becoming hard, A symptom saying that the liver is fighting to rid the body of whatever the result of taking MMS produces, dead bacteria or toxins. I think it might be wise if you mention a need for detoxing the liver or bowels as part of treatment with MMS.

A: I think if a person did a good job of detoxing his body before using MMS he might be more effective with a big dose. One girl tried this and it worked. She detoxed her body with liver detox and other methods for 2 months, and then in one day she took three 15 drops doses. That was 45 drops in one day at the very start of taking MMS. That was a hell of a MMS shock to the body, and it worked. She could tell within two days that her cancers were shrinking. She called me about it. She was ecstatic.

Should I lower my MMS dosage if I am feeling nauseous, tired and itchy?

Q: I have also been told many times of being weak in lymphatics and liver by naturopaths. Anyway I am wondering if I am doing the right thing. I am attempting to get up to 15 drops twice per day using raw apple cider vinegar, and maintain that for one week and then drop back to 6 drops. I am at 13 drops and feeling awful. It has taken me a week to get to this. I dread the drinking of it as it makes me want to vomit but I have only dry retched. I feel sluggish I feel tired I am itchy - indeed the first time I upped the dose to 4 drops my body broke out in hives for about one hour. Nauseous gastric pain do you think I should just go back down to 6 drops and should that be once or twice per day. It is hard to keep going

A: What you should do is reduce the amount of drops until

you quit feeling so bad. Maybe to 2 or 3 drops. Then begin taking more drops until you start feeling badly, and then reduce the drops until you no longer feel badly. Work your way up until you are taking 15 drops without feeling bad. However, do not stop taking them daily until you are OK at 15 drops daily. Then you can go to twice a week.

Will my liver have problems processing MMS if I have hepatitis C?

Q: I have hepatitis C and wonder if the liver will have problems processing this. Have you any advice or knowledge of hepatitis C sufferers recovering and totally clearing the virus?

A: I know of people with Hepatitis C and they say they feel much better after taking MMS. The liver should have no problems processing the supplement.

Will MMS help with cirrhosis of the liver, diabetes, and high blood pressure?

Q: I was told of you product and wanted to ask you if you thought my husband would be helped by taking it he has cirrhosis of the liver, diabetes, high blood pressure. I have started him on it cause I felt it could not hurt. I just wanted to know what you think. We are both taking it and I have a very dear friend who is taking it to help with her cancer.

A: Yes, I believe that the MMS will help all the conditions you mention. Just keep at it taking as much as you tolerate, but staying below the nausea level.

Is diarrhea an issue when someone's on immunosuppressive medicine?

Q: I am on an immunosuppressive medicine called Prograf for my Liver transplant. The liver is fine at the moment with lifelong prograf medicine. At present, I am planning to start MMS which will arrive today/tomorrow for my Ulcerative Colitis. I am taking Asacol, Prednisone 7.5mg, 125mcg Synthroid and 3 tablets Imodium a day. I am optimistic about MMS. The only concern is the immune system fight and the diarrhea control fight. I cannot control my diarrhea without Imodium. I hope you will reply.

A: Vomiting, Diarrhea are good indicators so do not worry about that just lower the dosage and you will be fine, if you are in any kind of medicine wait 4 hours when taking MMS, remember start at 1 drop per day and increase.

Is it safe to use MMS if I am also taking immunosuppressant drugs?

Q: I had a successful liver transplant in '05, but have Hep C that is attacking my new liver. I take the immunosuppressant Prograf so I do not reject my new organ. Do you think it's safe for me to use MMS?

A: Yes it is ok to take MMS. Just take it slowly; start at 1/2 drop per day and then gradually increase the dosage. Remember to stay beneath the point where it makes you feel nausea.

I have hepatitis C. Will my liver be able to process MMS?

Q: I have hepatitis C and wonder if the liver will have problems processing MMS. Have you any advice or knowledge of hepatitis C sufferers recovering and totally clearing the virus?

A: I know of people with Hepatitis C and they say they feel much better after taking MMS. The liver should have no problems processing the supplement.

Lungs

Do you think your product will help me improve my lungs condition?

Q: I had a kidney removed and lymphatic gland somewhere near my lungs, I am doing fine on wheat grass fruit and veggie diet, traces in my left kidney and lung have remained stable for a few years, do you think your product will help me get rid of it altogether?

A: I do not know if it will get rid of it all together but I think it will help you, give it a try and let me know how everything goes, if you have more questions let me know.

Lupus

Will MMS help me with my Lupus that I have been suffering from since 1986?

Q: Will MMS help me with my Lupus that I have been suffering from since 1986?

A: Everyone who has called me who has lupus all the

symptoms have disappeared, no one has ever reported negative reaction other than the standard normal reactions. There has been quite a few people reporting lupus symptoms all gone, as soon as the symptoms start disappearing you should get off the negative medicine.

Can MMS help me with Hepatitis C, Lupus and fungus nail problems?

Q: I have Hepatitis C and slightly elevated liver enzymes. I have Lupus and some fungus nail problems. I am a kidney dialysis patient. Can MMS help me with your formula?

A: All lupus cases so far have indicated that are gone, the viral count should reduce dramatically I do not know how long will it take, some people take longer than others. Anywhere to 2 weeks to 2 months take MMS so you can get ride off Hepatitis C.

Can I take MMS if I suffer from lupus?

Q: Can I take MMS if I suffer from lupus?

A: Yes everyone who has called me who has lupus all the symptoms have disappeared no one has ever reported negative reaction other than the standard normal reactions. There have been quite a few people reporting lupus symptoms all gone, as soon as the symptoms start disappearing you should get off the negative medicine.

Does MMS work well on lupus and other autoimmune diseases?

Q: Does MMS work well on lupus and other autoimmune diseases?

A: MMS works well with lupus and other autoimmune diseases. Many people with various autoimmune diseases have called to say they are OK.

Can I take MMS if I suffer from Lupus?

Q: Can I take MMS if I suffer from Lupus?

A: Yes, there have been quite a few people reporting that all their lupus symptoms have disappeared after adopting the MMS protocol. And no-one has ever reported negative reactions, other than the standard normal reactions.

As soon as the symptoms start disappearing, the patient should get off the negative medicine.

Lyme Disease

In the case of Lyme disease, has MMS caused severe die off?

Q: In the case of Lyme disease MMS has caused severe die off herxheimer reactions. When I first read part one of your book, the claim I read is that MMS renders all toxins inert. Clearly in the case of Lyme disease, IF toxins were rendered inert there would be no herxheimer reactions. I am assuming at this point that you are familiar with the term herx or herxheimer reaction which is when the Lyme bacteria is killed the dying bacteria

259

releases neurotoxins that cause flare ups to occur. This is also true of other bacteria I imagine.

A: I do not always get everything right. However, I do not remember saying all toxins, just most toxins. Maybe I did. Toxins that cause them selves to be eliminated from the body you do not have to worry about. They may make you sick for a while (called herxheimer reaction) but they do not stick around to do damage. The MMS probably would not do much damage to them. But that is not the poison that I am talking about. Poisons created by dead bacteria are not the same as poisons that inhibit the action of the body functions which are mostly heavy metals. The MMS seems to be able to oxidize them quite easily.

Do you think it would be OK to do 33 drops of MMS twice a day to rid Lyme Disease?

A: I suffer from Lyme disease and parasites. Do you think it would be OK to do 33 drops of MMS twice a day to rid my problem?

A: You could take 15 drops 4 times a day, however a better choice would be to do enemas, because the colon dumps the MMS into the plasma of the blood making it go deeper into the body to do enemas you should use 24 to 30 ounce of water and then use about the same dose as you would use by mouth and implanted in the colon that is put it in the colon and leave it if possible start at 4 or 5 drops of activated MMS and continue increasing by mouth. Do it 2 times a day.

Can MMS help my Lyme disease?

Q: I aim to use the product to eradicate my Lyme disease. Have you any real world experience with chronic Lyme? My friend Troy is undergoing EDTA chelation therapy in Dallas and is also taking DMSO intravenously. Do you know of any U.S. practitioners who administer MMS intravenously? Assuming that pharmaceutical grade product were available, would you have any hesitation about IV administration of MMS?

A: I am not sure that MMS IV will get the job done. Chelating and DMSO are not doing it either. MMS helps by mouth but it is not the answer. I have a Lyme case graveling to Mexico now and we will try a new protocol with MMS that I have high hopes of working to kill Lyme. If it works it will be fantastic and I will give the data to everyone just like MMS.

What do you recommend for a person who has been experiencing depression, irritability, brain fog and fatigue due to Lyme disease?

Q: I have Lyme disease and many of its co-infections; bartonella, babesia and ehrlichia, to name the big ones. I have been taking MMS for two weeks, but have only managed to get up to five drops, twice a day, because I am experiencing increased depression, irritability, brain fog and fatigue. (No nausea whatsoever though). I am tempted to ramp up faster per your instructions, but I fear the depression could get out of control. I am surprised that after two weeks, I only feel worse instead of better. My questions are: Has the same thing happened to other Lyme sufferers? What would you recommend as far as dosing? Do you think I could have detoxification problems and this is why I am not improving, or

261

is the MMS just killing a lot of bugs? Also, do you know if MMS can get Lyme in cystic form?

A: Most people who have Lyme disease have similar reactions, take less MMS keep the dose down to where you can tolerate it, the MMS Will handle most of the side disease and we are still working on a Lyme protocol other than what I am suggesting here, we are working and in my opinion you would have to go intervenes treatment before Lyme will be completely cured.

What would be the protocol for Lyme disease?

Q: Will MMS help me with my Lyme disease? What would be the protocol?

A: I have had many people with Lyme disease take MMS and it has helped them. Start at 10 drop an increase 1 drop a day, you can take it 2 or 3 times a day.

How many drops should I really need to take to get rid of Lyme disease coupled with Babesia?

Q: I have Lyme disease coupled with Babesia and who knows what other co-infections are probably raging in me. Can this really cure me? How many drops should I really need to take?

A: A lot of people that have contracted Lyme disease are taking MMS and it seems to help quite a bit but no one has said that there completely cured. I only have 2 people that have said they are cured. You must start out at 1 drop per day, you can take it 2 or 3 times a day, increase the drops 1 a day when you start getting nausea or get diarrhea lower the dosage, then when you get well keep increasing the drops until you get to 15 drops, There are a lot of people that take more than 15 drops but that depends on them. Everyone reacts differently.

Does MMS cross the brain blood barrier? Is it normal to have side effects from taking MMS after reaching 15 drops a day?

Q: Does MMS cross the brain blood barrier? I have Lyme disease and I am starting to feel the neurological problems. I started three days ago on MMS and was not getting any side effects but felt great and clear headed then I got up to 15 drops a day and started getting diarrhea and nausea and aching joints. Do you have any suggestions?

A: Most people who have Lyme have similar reactions, take less MMS keep the dose down to where you can tolerate it.

We are still working on a Lyme disease protocol other than what I am suggesting here we are working and in my opinion you would have to get MMS through and IV before Lyme will be completely handled.

How long do I need to take MMS to complete a treatment for Lyme disease?

Q: I am currently using MMS. I am on my second day of 15 drops once a day. How long do I need to take it to complete treatment for Lyme disease?

A: Take MMS at 15 drops 2 times a day for two weeks and

then lower the dose to 6 drops a day which is the maintenance dose. So far the most effective way is 3 or 4 drops three or 4 times a day.

Does stabilized oxygen work with MMS? Will this formula help with Endogenous Retroviruses and Lyme Disease?

Q: Is the Stabilized Oxygen OK to use with the vinegar/juice formula? It has deionized water, potassium Chlorite and sodium bicarbonate? Will this formula help with Endogenous Retroviruses? Will MMS also help get rid of my Lyme disease?

A: Stabilized oxygen does not work with MMS, it will not create the chlorine dioxide, as far as Lyme disease is concern it should help you, I think that enemas are the most effective way against it. Flush the colon out first with water and aloe vera or a teaspoon or two of baking soda. Then flush out the baking soda. Then implant the MMS just as if it were a dose to be taken by mouth. Keep increasing the drops until you reach at least 16 drops per implant. Leave it in as long as possible. It should all be absorb into the sides of the colon.

What dose of MMS would you recommend for Lyme disease?

Q: What dose of MMS would you recommend for Lyme disease?

A: So far the most effective way is 3 or 4 drops 3 or 4 times a day. A lot of people with Lyme disease have taken MMS and it seems to help quite a bit but no one has said that there

264

completely cure, only 2 people have said they are cured.

Can you let me know how to make the 10% citric acid solution and the procedure on the IV approach to treat Lyme Disease patients?

Q: I like the idea of smaller doses more often as the stomach is often compromised with Lyme patients. However, I would like to know how to make the 10% citric acid solution and the procedure on the IV approach.

A: I do not think that Lyme patients are going to start getting well until the IV approach is used. From what I have seen so far in one patient, I am convinced that is what is going to be necessary.

Would MMS work on borreliosis (Lyme Disease), meningitis, multiple sclerosis and aphtas?

Q: I have just three questions about MMS, Did you make experience with tick bites and tick fever (borreliosis and meningitis)? Is there also an effect with multiple sclerosis? What do you think about aphtas in the mouth?

A: It helps for ticks, there has been some people who have reported good results.

Q2. Several people who have MS have reported that they have overcome all or almost all of their symptoms and that they have their life back. I cannot promise you anything, and I certainly would not say that I know for sure that it cures anything; but a hundred thousand people so far, have reported being well or a lot better. If they remain cured? I do not know. Not enough time has passed since the reports of those who said they are back to their life. At this time, I can say that MMS has a record for more people becoming well than any other substance.

Q3. MMS works for apthas, in fact, people have reported they have recovered. It should be noted that MMS helps for almost everything concerning oral hygiene and it does make the mouth a lot healthier.

Is there a way to take Vitamin C without affecting my MMS treatment?

Q: I began MMS then the Vitamin C and salt protocol that has had a beneficial effect on me. How can I do both, as it is not good to take Vitamin C with MMS?. My lyme disease is mostly severe fatigue brain fog and altered vision. If you have an insight please let me know. I changed my protocol from 6 at 8pm then 6 at 9pm to 4 in the morning and 4 at 8 and 9 pm after a slow progression. I do not know how to coordinate Vitamin C/salt with MMS every hours for my eyes. (the Vitamin C/ salt obviously improved my energy but does not help my eyes.

A: Just separate vitamin C and MMS by four hours. In this regard, you are going to have to work it out somehow. Also you might try enemas for more results with lyme.

What is the protocol for taking MMS for Lyme disease and severe CFIDS?

Q: I have very severe CFIDS (chronic fatigue and immune dysfunction syndrome), and I am totally bedridden much of the time. Several doctors feel I may also have late stage Lyme disease as well as metals.

I did not tolerate 3 months of antibiotics at all. Can MMS help me? I started MMS treatment two nights ago. I put 2 drops in a cup, mixed 1/2 teaspoon of lime juice. Waited for 3 minutes. Added 1/3 cup of water. I want to make sure I am doing this right.

It seems like MMS also kills many bacteria. Can MMS eradicate viruses and bacteria that hide out in cells and replicate in ways that the immune system does not find them?

A: For every drop of MMS you need to add 5 drops of citric acid, lime or lemon juice, wait 3 minutes and then add half a glass of water or juice.

The most effective way that I have found to help eradicate Lyme disease so far is to take 3 or 4 drops, 3 or 4 times a day.

A lot of people who have Lyme disease have taken MMS and it seems to help quite a bit, but no one has reported back to me that they are completely cured yet.

I personally had people tested for heavy metals before and after taking MMS and the heavy metals were totally reduced after 2 weeks.

Malaria

I have Malaria, but not the full blown malaria, what do you suggest I take?

Q: I have the malaria that keeps recurring, my liver and spleen are suffering. Should I do shock treatment even though I do not have full blown malaria? Also I am bleeding from the rectum. is that ok? How long will the vomiting, diarrhea and bleeding last?

A: To avoid nausea, try 5 drops at 1 hour intervals for fifteen drops in the morning and 15 drops in the afternoon in the same way. That will probably do the job; if it does not you will have to shock it. I would stop using MMS until the bleeding and diarrhea and vomiting stops. I assume that you did what was suggested. If you did anything else let me know. After those symptoms stop you should start back at 1 drop and work up to more drops slowly.

What is the dosage for people with Malaria?

Q: The MMS just arrived here today. After I return from Alexandria in four or five days, I will start treating two people with malaria right here in Cairo. Sudanese nationals. Then in a week or so after that, I will head down to the border and treat a few people there. I will start out with 18 drops . If that makes them vomit then I will go down to 6 drops every hour for 4 hours as you prescribed in your email below. How long does it take to clear the patient from malaria? I assume that is relative to the degree of infection, am I right ? I need to know this, because I know I am going to be asked how long will it take to eliminate malaria. What's the best and the worse case scenario, as far as time scale for clearing a person of malaria ? Do I also give children 6 drops hourly for 4 hours? When you have time, give me whatever info you can on how to determine the amount and frequency of drops / dosages. I am going to go to your book in the meantime, and see if I can get info on this.

A: 90% of the cases of malaria will be free of malaria with all symptoms gone in 4 hours. It will look like miracles. You just have to do it right. Use 15 to 18 drops depending upon the person the bigger the person the more drops, but do not go over 18 drops for the first dose or under 15 for smaller persons. Then in one to 4 hours give the second dose. Normally the first dose cures the malaria and the second dose goes deeper to kill the remaining. Remember, all doses require the lemon juice or citric acid, 5 drops for each 1 drop of MMS, wait three minutes and add the juice. I always provided pineapple juice, about 1/2 glass and I often diluted the pineapple juice with 50% water to make it go further. Children use less. For malaria judge their size and weight but it should be 3 drops for each 25 pounds (11.4 kg) of body weight. When you have a long line of kids, you do not have time to weigh them. Just judge their weight. Just error on the side of too much MMS rather than too little. If only a few people vomit. Do not change the doses. Only change if most people are vomiting. Judge these things correctly as when other people see someone vomiting they will refuse to take the stuff. There is a lot of data and instructions in the above paragraph. Please read it a few times.

Multiple Sclerosis

Is MS an autoimmune diseases?

Q: I read the story of MS patient who experienced many symptoms in her body were gone. I noticed that she/he? is claiming that MS is a autoimmune disease. And I feel that Parkinson also could be the same category…. immune cells were attacking the neurons in substantia nigra. If this theory is right…. Do you think MMS would help Parkinson's patient also? Is there any example(s) of the recovery (full or half)with Parkinson's by drinking MMS solutions?

A: I have not known of any person just yet, but you would be surprised how many people have been cured from other diseases. Give it a try and let me know how it goes.

Will MMS help with my Multiple Sclerosis (MS)?

Q: Will this help with my Multiple Sclerosis (MS)?

A: Several people who have MS have reported to me that they have overcome all or almost all of their symptoms and that they have their life back. I cannot promise you anything and I certainly would not say that I know for sure that it cures MS. But a hundred thousand people so far have reported being well and feeling lot better. Not enough time has passed since the reports of those who said they are back to their life. At this time I can say that MMS has a record for more people becoming well than any other substance.

Can MMS help me with my Multiple Sclerosis (MS) and

Tuberculosis(TB)?

Q: Can MMS help me with my MS and TB?

A: We have had good results with TB and with MS. It takes a while for MS, TB is faster, but both take a bit of time.

Can MMS help get rid of Multiple Sclerosis?

Q: We have heavy pathogen loads which are depriving our bodies of nutrients needed to heal. For some reason we also all seem to have heavy metal loads like Mercury, Lead, cadmium, arsenic. I do not know if anyone contaminant occurred first or what brought on our susceptibility but I believe people who have MS should take the MMS very slowly. I am still at 3 drops 3 times a day and continue to have headaches with a little queasiness and small pains in stomach. Others on the board are also experiencing this as well at low doses. Is there any remedy for the headache or queasiness that is compatible with the MMS? How long does this response last? In the letter you sent about immune disease cures can you elaborate and say what diseases you are speaking about?

A: So far there are only a couple of MS people reporting feeling a lot better, but there is not enough time to tell how long it takes to get rid of the viral load. However, most of the heavy metals should be gone within two weeks. MMS is real fast with many things, even fast with MS but there is a lot of things to handle. MMS is only an oxidizer. The body then handles the repair of the damage and/or healing. There is no nutritional value in MMS. It just kills the bad stuff. So the answer is: we do not yet know how long the headaches will last. It they get too bad, drop back to less drops. If it gets really bad, cancel the MMS by drinking a glass of water with 2000 mg of Vitamin C crystals dissolved in it. About the headaches. Lay down on a bed or couch, relax the body, and then concentrate on relaxing the tension within the head. Do it right, and the headache is gone. There are a few herbs that help. The local health food store might know.

Will MMS work for Multiple Sclerosis (MS), Breast cancer, Psoriasis or Eczema?

Q: I was wondering if MMS will work for Multiple Sclerosis and breast cancer. Has anybody written to you about using it for MS or after cancer maintenance? Have you found that it also works for Psoriasis or Eczema?

A: Several people who have MS have reported to me that they have overcome all or almost all of their symptoms and that they have their life back. I cannot promise you anything and I certainly would not say that I know for sure that it cures anything. But a hundred thousand people so far have reported being well or a lot better. If it stays cured I do not know. Not enough time has passed since the reports of those who said they are back to their life. At this time I can say that MMS has a record for more people becoming well than any other substance. When a person is taking any kind of drug always let a 4 hour period wait until taking MMS.

Do you have some cases in which patients with Chronic Fatigue were healed with MMS?

Q: My wife has chronic fatigue and my mother-in-law has

272

multiple sclerosis. Do you have some cases that patients with this condition were healed with MMS?

A: I do have some success stories for chronic fatigue but I would have to ask people for permission in order to pass it around, for MS Several people who have MS have reported to me that they have overcome all or almost all of their symptoms and that they have their life back.

Can this help someone with pancreatic cancer who just started chemo, having had spleen, gull bladder and the tumor in the pancreas removed as well as degenerative MS?

Q: Can this help someone with pancreatic cancer who just started chemo, having had spleen, gull bladder and the tumor in the pancreas removed? Have you had any results with degenerative ms?

A: For the cancer follow the cancer protocol and for Multiple sclerosis start with the standard protocol.

Will MMS help with my Multiple Sclerosis?

Q: Will this help with my multiple sclerosis?

A: Several people who have MS have reported to me that they have overcome all or almost all of their symptoms. I cannot promise you anything and I certainly would not say that I know for sure that it cures MS. But a hundred thousand people so far have reported feeling a lot better. At this time I can say that MMS has a record for more people becoming well than any other substance.

Nausea and Stomach

Is there anything I could do to overcome revulsion towards the taste and smell of MMS?

Q: I have been taking MMS now for about 6 months, at least 5 X week. I worked up to a therapeutic dose of just 13 drops when I had vomiting/diarrhea, so I stayed there for 10 days, and had been on a maintenance dose of 6-8 drops per day. 4 weeks ago I came down with a severe congestion in my chest; no cold or sore throat, did have body aches and fever the first two days. I have been taking MMS 2-4 X day, up to 40 drops total per day, and I still have the congestion with coughing up thick yellow-green phlegm; no fever/body aches. I thought I was over it twice and discontinued the MMS for 2 days each time, but the congestion returned.

I just read your site and realize perhaps I should take smaller doses more often throughout the day and do not skip any days. But, I can hardly stand taking the MMS anymore the smell alone makes my whole body spasm in revulsion which seems like my body is saying "NO MORE!". Please advice?

A: Many people seem to get the revulsion of MMS. The best answer I have found so far is to buy some frozen concentrated dark grape juice. Then do not add the full amount of water. Add about 1/4 less water. That makes a strong grape juice. That will usually hide the entire taste of the MMS. Try it. If you still have a little problem, add two teaspoons of citric acid solution to the grape juice just before you drink it.

I have also found that as the body gets cleaned out of microorganisms that it becomes more and more tolerant of the MMS chlorine dioxide. I think that some of the more intelligent organisms can create the revulsion. It's not the body, but the guys that are fighting to stay causing their havoc. Yes, the smaller doses but more often seems to get the best results. I once had the revulsion but I kept at it and now with the grape juice even without the stronger grape juice I taste noting and I can tolerate very high doses without revulsion. Same with many other people.

Have you heard of acid reflux occurring from someone taking MMS?

Q: Have you heard of acid reflux occurring from someone taking MMS? She took a single drop, and does not know what might have caused the reaction. She said that she noted an improvement in her sinuses, and she also notices increased energy… but the acid reflux is troubling. Any insights or suggestions that you have will be most appreciated.

A: This sort of reaction often happens from MMS. Many problems often turn back on for a few days or a few hours when taking MMS. The reason for this is that when many problems seem to disappear, especially from drugs or other treatments, it is because they are covered over. They have not been cured; they have been covered over or pushed deeper into the system. MMS destroys the things that cover the problems and the problems reappear. But if you continue, they will disappear. Normally it is worth the time to overcome and destroy these things as you are cleaning your body. Again, normally, if you do not destroy these things they will reappear later in life. And normally, with MMS they only reappear for a few hours, sometimes for a few days, but usually it is not very long.

Meanwhile, baking soda is the best thing to use when the acid feeling begins. A level teaspoon should be enough. Put it in 1/4 glass of water. But do not use the baking soda until the acid feeling starts and that should be at least an hour after taking the MMS. If you use the baking soda right away after taking the MMS you will neutralize the MMS and thus get no benefit.

Do you have any suggestions for the nausea I have been experiencing?

Q: My husband has type 1 diabetes and suffered a mild heart attack about 4 weeks ago he has had many complications due to the diabetes so we are hoping to see some results, I myself was diagnosed with diverticulitis and both of us suffer with nail rot. We have started at 7 drops with citric acid, I am on 10 and my husband on 9 so far I have been experiencing nausea and very tired. Would you have any suggestions?

A: If you are experiencing nausea, you should drop back a few drops until you do not feel nauseous. It will be easier for you. It might take a little longer, but not much.

Does not feeling any nausea mean that MMS is not working?

Q: Never felt any nausea. Is it a good/bad sign? Does it not mean that MMS is unable to find any bad stuff in the body to oxidize?

A: It is normal for someone to not experience any nausea, vomiting or diarrhea. Just wait until you get to 15 drops 3 times a day. And you are right, there was very little to oxidize but that does not mean that some very dangerous pathogens were not killed.

How long can someone stay on 15 drops of MMS once a day?

Q: How do I know how long to take MMS after I reach 15 drops once a day? I have had parasites due to a bird mite infestation and want to strengthen my immune system. I also have high cholesterol so I want to take it for that. I am up to 9 drops and am experiencing diarrhea and stomach cramping. I know it says this is a normal reaction, but should I continue increasing the dosage?

A: When you experience diarrhea, nausea or vomiting just lower the dose to 1 or 2 drops. When this stops, starts increasing the dose again, until you get past that sickness.

Stay 1 week at 15 drops (if you are well you can take it 2 or 3 times a day.) After that week stay at the maintenance dose of 4 or 6 drops a day for older people and 4 to 6 drops twice a week for younger people.

Why Does MMS Cause Burping and Strange After Taste?

Q: There is a lot of positive effects happening with the MMS. I am currently at 12 drops twice a day and experiencing mild nausea but burping what tastes like blood for a couple hours. I am taking the drops after eating. So my question is can MMS cause ulcers or stomach problems? Any other thoughts you have that my help my road to wellness would be appreciated.

A: MMS has never caused stomach problems so far, and certainly not ulcers. However, it does kill growths in the stomach and other colonies of microorganisms. This could be the cause of the taste of blood, but it is only something that needs to be killed as MMS cannot kill beneficial organisms or healthy cells. Taking MMS is often killing microorganisms or larger organisms that are not causing problems in the present, but that will cause problems 10 or 20 years down the road. MMS has no food value at all to cause any kind of problem. It cannot kill beneficial body parts or organisms as it is a very weak oxidizer.

Pacemaker

Can MMS be taking with a medicine called Warfarin?

Q: Sorry to trouble you again about my question on MMS with taking Warfarin. Maybe I missed your reply somehow. You were going to look into the pacemaker side of taking this product.

A: I do not have any information on warfarin, however no one has reported problems with a pacemaker. It should not bother a pacemaker as it does not have the power to react with metals; especially those used in the body, and of course, plastics it does not react with. (Except, of course, heavy metals that are in the chemical form.) My suggestion so far has been to start with tiny doses and work up. Start with 1/2 drop mixed with 2.5 drops of lemon or citric acid solution (10%). Use a small glass; tip the glass on the side, put in one drop. Add 5 drops of the lemon or citric and wait 3 minutes, then add one half glass of water. Now's the trick. Dump 1/2 of that out, and you now have 1/2 drop in solution.

Can an 87 year old man with a pacemaker and on blood thinners take MMS?

Q: Is it possible for an 87 year old man with a pacemaker and on blood thinners to take MMS?

A: Yes, it is possible, just start out very slowly. I start with 1/2 drop the first day. Look for negative effects, and then go to 1 drop. Negative effects do not mean that there is a problem because killing pathogens creates poisons in the system. But if you notice a problem with the pacemaker do not increase, but do not stop. The MMS does not affect metals and other items. It only kills the pathogens. Just go slow.

Pancreas

Can a person with 2 organ transplants and on dialysis take MMS?

Q: I am inquiring for one of our customers: Her question: Her son has had 2 organ transplants in the past few years. One was and kidney, the other a pancreas. He has other heart issues due to the transplants and dialysis. She wants to know if taking the MMS would be harmful to him or in your opinion, would it be ok for him to take it.

A: In my opinion the MMS would help. The reason I believe this is that in many different autoimmune diseases, the MMS stopped the disease. This might stump you as it seem that increasing the power of the immune system would just give it that much more power to attack the body, but that does not happen. The reason being, again in my opinion is that all disorders of the body is caused by microorganisms that are in some way growing in the body. MMS kills all such microorganisms. So far no one has indicated a problem with using MMS with transplants. However, I would go very slowly just to be cautious and safe. Start out at 1/2 drop MMS dose. Make a one drop dose and pour out 1/2 of it. Take a 1/2 dose every day for a weeks or so.

Does MMS cure diabetes?

Q: What about diabetes, does MMS cure diabetes?

A: A group of researchers in Canada have stated that all persons with diabetes have an inflamed pancreas. Many doctors have said that, so it's really nothing new. What is new is MMS. The Chlorine Dioxide created by the MMS overcomes the inflammation of the pancreas and guess what, the symptoms of the diabetes.

Can this help someone with pancreatic cancer who just started chemo, having had spleen, gull bladder and the tumor in the pancreas removed as well as degenerative MS?

Q: Can this help someone with pancreatic cancer who just started chemo, having had spleen, gull bladder and the tumor in the pancreas removed? Have you had any results with degenerative Ms?

A: For the cancer follow the cancer protocol and for Multiple sclerosis start with the standard protocol.

What is the recommendation to start MMS treatment on a patient with pancreatic cancer?

Q: My father is currently battling pancreatic cancer Stage IV. He has just been administered his fifth treatment of Chemotherapy, and although it MAY be slowing it down, it is still advancing. My main question for you is this: What have been your experiences with pancreatic cancer? Do you recommend a certain starting point or should we begin and do 1/2 drop to begin with and work up from there?

A: A number of people have called to say that they were succeeding with pancreatic cancer. Starting with 1/2 drop would be the best.

I am wondering whether the mechanism on diabetes is microbe or metal related?

Q: I am wondering what the mechanism might be on diabetes? Would it mean diabetes might be microbe related in some cases? Or, metal related?

A: Generally, what is involved with the diabetes is the pancreas being inflamed; MMS gets the inflammation down, thus the pancreas starts working again. However, it is not a solution for everybody, and only half of the people taking MMS have been helped. If the inflammation goes down the problem might be microbe related.

Parasites

Since I am pregnant, Is the six drop dosage powerful enough to kill worms?

Q: I am breastfeeding my one year old child. A friend of my husband told us about your product MMS and wrote to you about whether it is safe to take while breastfeeding. You said it was safe, but to limit it to the 6 drop dosage. I believe I can feel parasites / worms moving around inside of me and have seen my waste moving around in the toilet. I think my two daughters may have parasites / worms too. On the bottle of MMS, it says that the 15 drop dosage should be used to kill parasites / worms. My questions are:

1. Is the six drop dosage powerful enough to kill the worms or should I be doing something else? Should I take a drug to kill the worms and then take your product? Also, is the child and baby dosages strong enough to kill the worms in the kids?

2. Can I take the 6 drop dosage and give the baby dosage to my one year old (breastfeeding) daughter at the same time?

3. My 5 year old daughter, husband, and I have been taking MMS for 4 days. We are up to 4 drops once a day, taking one extra drop each day. How many times a day should we be taking MMS?

A: Go for 15 to kill the worms, But go slowly working up to that does one drop at a time. You can take the MMS from one to three times a day. Look at how you feel and how much you think you can take without making yourself too nauseous. It is good for babies, but if the baby becomes nauseous you might have to use a bottle for a few days, not likely, but maybe. If the 3 drops for 25 pounds of body weight does not do it, use more.

Does MMS kill or eliminate Candida and parasites?

Q: Does MMS kill or eliminate Candida? Does MMS kill or eliminate parasites?

A: Yes MMS will help with Candida and parasites, just take MMS with citric acid, lime or lemon.

Is MMS effective against parasites?

Q: I was wondering if MMS is effective against parasites?

A: Yes I have people that have told me that MMS has helped them rid their parasites after taking MMS.

Is it OK to take 1/2 a drop of MMS to eliminate bacteria and parasites?

Q: Is it possible that the bacteria and parasites can grow faster than what MMS can clean? Or can I take for a long time 1/2 drop and the body cleans with that little?

A: I think you should keep up with the 1/2 drop for a while.

You will eventually go past that drop. Diarrhea is a good indicator, that means that your body is eliminating bad pathogens. However, do not allow yourself to continue with diarrhea. Be sure to take less drops. If you get too tired, just take MMS when you go to bed.

Parkinson's Disease

Can MMS help Parkinson's Disease?

Q: My husband has bladder cancer and diverticulitis. I have Parkinson's disease. We have both been taking MMS for a couple of months now. I know that MMS helps cancer however is there any cases known that it helps Parkinson's or if not do you feel that it can help?

A: I had several people that told me MMS has helped them with Parkinson, I think it will help but no one has told me that they have been cured yet. I believe that it may be necessary to take MMS by IV infusion or enemas to make a big difference. I have good reports for a lot of disease that they are reporting and many are being cured but none that I am aware of for Parkinson's disease.

Are there any cases where MMS has helped Parkinson's disease?

Q: My husband has bladder cancer and diverticulitis.

I have Parkinson's disease. We have both been taking MMS for a couple of months now. I have ordered your book.

I know that MMS helps cancer, however are there any known cases of MMS helping Parkinson's disease. If not, do you feel that it can help?

A: I have heard from several people that MMS has helped them with Parkinson's disease. I think MMS will help but no-one has told me that they have been cured yet.

I believe that it may be necessary to take MMS by IV infusion or enemas to make a big difference.

I have good reports from many people that they are being cured of many different diseases but so far I have not received any reports from people with Parkinson's disease that they have been totally cured through the use of MMS.

Pathogens

How many electrons are accepted when chlorine dioxide comes into contact?

Q: I am just curious. Which is correct? Four (4) or five (5) electrons are accepted/taken when chlorine dioxide comes into contact with a pathogen?

A: The correct amount is five electrons.

Is it really necessary to max the dose of MMS as quickly as possible?

Q: Do you use the MMS on a daily dosage for yourself? If so how long have you used your current dose. I need to know your opinion on how I am treating my MS. I believe MS is triggered by many pathogens. I am maintaining interest in the MMS treatment and am making progress. I do not know what to expect will happen but due to the severity of my disease I have chosen to use lower strength and more doses per day. I want to build slowly so I do not have severe herx or headaches as that is too fatiguing for me. I read you suggest to go to the max dose as quickly as possible. I would like to know with the problems I have described is that necessary? I am not getting much queeziness or nausea.

A: You are doing very well. Four or 5 times a day is best. Just keep it up. If you feel like increasing the drops each time do so, and if you feel queasy do not increase, back off a drop or so. Just keep at it.

What toxins are washed away from the body using your MMS solution?

Q: What toxins are washed away from the body using your MMS solution?

A: MMS kills pathogens and oxidizes heavy metals, the body then washes away the residue. There is some evidence that MMS oxidizes other toxins, but I do not know which ones. However, what most people believe is caused by toxins is almost always caused by pathogens, often colonies of pathogens that are not known, but when they are killed many problems disappear.

How does MMS kill the bacteria?

Q: If the MMS kills bacteria, how does it deal with the body's natural bacteria which consists of 80% good and 20% bad? I know you state that it leaves healthy cells and kills the harmful ones, but can it differentiate between bacteria and leave the body's natural bacteria (good and bad) alone? If all the bacteria is destroyed are you promoting a probiotic?

A: Good bacteria in the body are known as aerobic bacteria (that means that they use oxygen). Disease causing bacteria are Anaerobic (that means they do not use oxygen). You might suppose then, that there is some sort of difference between them and that is true, there is a difference. Guess what, the unique qualities of the MMS ion (chlorine dioxide) allows it to see the difference between the two different bacteria, and thus it only destroys the anaerobic bacteria (that's the disease causing bacteria). This is also controlled by the white blood cells in the immune system which have the ability to use chlorine dioxide against the diseases.

Respiratory Conditions

Does MMS help overcome Asthma?

Q: Does MMS help overcome Asthma?

A: MMS has often stopped an asthma attack in 10 minutes or less, but it does not work every time. MMS works best with asthma over a longer period of time. It depends upon the condition of the asthma whether or not it stops an attack instantly or how long it takes to overcome a condition of asthma. MMS will always help, but if a person is "beyond repair," then MMS will not do the job. However, "Beyond repair" is seldom the case and over a period of time it will often handle the asthma.

Start with two drops twice a day for the first day, taking the drops after a meal. If the person gets nauseous he will often stop taking the solution and refuse to take more so be careful to avoid making someone nauseous. In any case, work up to 15 drops 3 times a day. It may take months before one can do this without being nauseous. This is because the MMS is slowly destroying something and is bringing about detoxification of the body. (That's what I think, but the fact is I have watched many people get well from various diseases and they usually are well and feeling energetic when the drops are no longer causing nausea.) Asthma is not easy to clear up, but it has cleared up in those who kept with it.

Several days ago (1/4/2008), a lady called to say that all asthma symptoms were totally gone. She said that she called me two months before this and stated that her asthma symptom had gotten much worse since she started taking MMS. She said that she went from 6 times using the inhaler to using it 12 times a day. But when I told her not to stop, she said that she would not and in fact she did not stop even though her asthma remained worse for a month and a half. Then all of a sudden it started getting better. In less than 15 days it decreased to not needing the inhaler at all and breathing totally easy.

Does MMS help overcome Asthma?

Q: Does MMS help overcome Asthma?

A: Start with two drops twice a day for the first day, taking the drops after a meal. If the person gets nauseous he will often stop taking the solution and refuse to take more so be careful to avoid making someone nauseous. In any case, work up to 15 drops 3 times a day. It may take months before one can do this without being nauseous. This is because the MMS is slowly destroying something and is bringing about detoxification of the body. (That's what I think, but the fact is I have watched many people get well from various diseases and they usually are well and feeling energetic when the drops are no longer causing nausea.) Asthma is not easy to clear up, but it has cleared up in those who kept with it.

How long do you think it will be before I can see some results from using MMS?

Q: I wonder if you would be good enough to give me some feedback now that I have started taking the MMS. I suffer from a respiratory condition where my lungs and sinuses are badly affected. As a result of years of ongoing suffering I have developed very bad nasal polyps. Usually the inhaler I use gives me some lung relief. Now that I have started taking the MMS I am not getting that relief any more and my body is starting to tremble slightly. My condition is suddenly much worse and I am hoping this is all on account of taking the MMS.

I have not suffered any nausea, but my condition is accentuated all the same. I wonder if this is just another manifestation of nausea. I have backed off on the dosage which was 15 drops X 2 twice daily as advised in your book for people who are sick. I know I cannot be accurately diagnosed, but in your opinion do you think the MMS is working and how long do you think it will be before I can see some results from it? I am into my fourth day of taking the MMS.

A: Fifteen drops twice a day is 10 times too much to start off with. Please quit that amount immediately. Go to maybe 3 drops twice a day until you are feeling at least back to normal. That might take two weeks. Then start to increase the drops slowly. Wow. Easy does it!

What experiences have you had with Emphysema?

Q: What experiences have you had with Emphysema?

A: We have had several people write and call to let us know that they have been doing much better from emphysema after taking MMS.

Will MMS help with Allergic Bronchial Aspergillosis?

Q: Will MMS help with Allergic Bronchial Aspergillosis?

A: MMS has been use for a lot of disease, but not all the people that take MMS let me know if it has helped them. I am sure it will help you with your problem.

Would MMS help combat a bacterial infection in the sinuses and Candida?

Q: I was about to start the MMS protocol for my Candida problem, when I came down with a bacterial infection in my left maxillary sinus. Would MMS help combat a bacterial infection in the sinuses as well?

A: Yes it will help you. Just use the standard protocol.

Can MMS be used with a mist generator to help me breath better?

Q: My nasal cavity is completely blocked and there is no way in or out regarding any substances or air. I am literally drowning in my own discolored mucus. So I will have to rely on your second suggestion and that is to breathe it. I have found a mist generator that is used for greenhouses and around ponds. Is this the same machine? If so can you advise me on how to use it? Also please advise on the kind of solution I use for the generator. In the beginning I will only be able to breathe it through my mouth, but I am hoping the polyposis will be addressed by taking the MMS formula orally.

A: Yes, and be sure to gargle with it two or three times a day. Make a 6 drop dose, add the water, and gargle with it. Even four times a day. Remember that 6 drops of MMS, 30 of citric acid solution, wait three minutes, then add half a glass of water. You may use a standard glass, although this is not critical.

Will it help if I rinse my face with a solution of MMS in hopes of preventing the continued appearance of those precancerous keratoses?

Q: I was wondering was the efficacy or rinsing my face with a solution in hopes of preventing the continued appearance of those precancerous keratoses, or the disappearance of those that are already there.... Has anyone tried a mild solution in a small volume neutralizer for chronic asthma? Or will the

291

internal solution help?

A: Get a small spray 2 ounce bottle mix 20 drops of MMS with 100 drops of citric acid solution, or lemon juice, wait 3 minutes and fill the rest of the 2 ounce bottle with water, spray it on 2 or 3 times a day and keep taking MMS by mouth. If the spray stings, then reduce the strength by pouring out ½ of the bottle and adding water. It can help asthma and so will taking it by mouth. Most asthma sufferers get relief and over time seem to be cured. The spray is a different strength than taking it by mouth.

Skin

Do I have to wash the solution off my skin after a certain time if I am applying it topically?

Q: I am currently at 15 drops three times per day and feeling ok apart from some tiredness and a slight headache. I am using the MMS at the rate prescribed for the warts topically - 3 drops MMS with 15 drops of citric acid waiting 3 minutes and applying directly to the wart by cotton bud..some burning sensation is there for about an hour and after 3 days some redness is evident surrounding the warts..my question is do I wash the solution off after a certain time or do i leave it on straight..I am doing the same protocol as for the insect bites

A: I do not know where you got the 3 drops from, I always suggest when using topically get 2 ounce spray bottle and use 20 drops of MMS and 100 drops of citric acid wait 3 minutes and add it to the 2 ounce bottle and add water to that and spray it on. If you feel a burning sensation wash it off and in a couple of minutes spray some again.

Can MMS be used topically for skin ailments and rashes?

Q: Can MMS be used topically ? I was thinking of adding it to my clay mask...which i mix with a little apple cider vinegar and the clay powder bentonite and apply as in a facial or to other parts of the body... but I was thinking, could it be used in the same way for skin ailments, rashes and such?(antioxidants are antioxidants - they can be introduced topically to heal the skin, as well as internally, yes ?). What has been your experience and recommendation with this ?

A: Seems like it should work, but my experience is that it does not. It is not an antioxidant. It is a powerful oxidizer. The best experience I have had so is to use MMS as a spray for the skin. It kills pathogens on the skin and overcome all kinds of infections. Use 20 drops of MMS in a 2 ounce bottle. Activate that with 100 drops of citric acid mixture or lemon juice, wait three minutes and then fill the bottle with water. That mixture at that strength will last 3 days. Use that to spray on any skin problem two to four times a day. Let it dry on the skin. Rinse it off once before bed, let it dry and spray it again. If it hurts or burns at any time rinse it off.

Is MMS ever used topically for toenails or dry spots or melanoma spots?

Q: Is it ever used topically for toenails or dry spots or melanoma spots?

A: Yes it has been used topically, what you can do is put it directly on your toe, what I suggest is putting it directly on the toe with the fungus mix for example 6 drops of MMS with 30 of citric acid and a table spoon of water and splash it on your toes you can leave it there over night or a few hours and just rinse it. For the melanoma spots take a 2 ounce bottle and mix 20 drop of MMS and 100 drops of citric acid solution wait 3 minutes and fill the rest of the 2 ounce bottle with water, spray it on your melanoma 2 or 3 times a day and keep taking MMS by mouth.

Will MMS help me with a break out of pimples I have all over both hands and the insides of my forearms?

Q: I had surgery to fix hernias and when I got out of hospital my hands started itching and breaking out with pimples and it has spread all over both hands and the insides of my forearms. I have tried everything and the doctors do not help. Will this help me? Also during my surgery or after my kidneys shut down, after a strong water pill and walking I was able to urinate normally again, but I feel this could be connected?

A: Take a 12 ounce bottle put 20 drops and 100 drops of citric acid wait 3 minutes add the water and the mixture to the bottle and spray it on the affected area, also you should start taking it by mouth start the standard protocol.

Will MMS help me with psoriasis?

Q: I have had psoriasis for years now. Will MMS help me? How much should I take?

A: MMS will help you with your psoriasis you start by taking one drop and five drops of citric acid twice a day and increasing the dose daily. The goal is to get up to 15 drops and then go back to a maintenance level of 6 drops.

Will MMS remove all types of wart viruses and what dosage and for how long should I use it? Also does it work on the HPV viruses?

Q: Will MMS remove all types of wart viruses and what dosage and for how long should I use it? Also does it work on the HPV viruses?

A: MMS has killed so many viruses, just start with the standard protocol, go to my website and under important information you will find the standard protocol.

What is the best to cure Varicose Eczema?

Q: What is the best to cure Varicose Eczema?

A: Start at 1 drop per day, you can take it 2 or 3 times a day, next day take 2 drops and so on until you get to 15 drops. If you get diarrhea or nausea back off 1 drop until you feel better. Then you increase the drops again.

How much MMS shall I take to treat my Psoriasis?

Q: I have had psoriasis for years now. Will MMS help me? How much shall I take?

A: MMS will help you with your psoriasis you start by taking one drop and five drops of citric acid twice a day and increasing the dose daily. The goal is to get up to 15 drops and then go back to a maintenance level of 6 drops.

Will MMS help me treat a skin breakout?

Q: I had surgery to fix hernias and when I got out of hospital my hands started itching and breaking out with bad pimples and it has spread all over both hands and the insides of my forearms. I have tried everything and the doctors do not help. Will this help me?

A: Take a 2 ounce bottle put 20 drops and 100 drops of citric acid wait 3 minutes add the water and the mixture to the bottle and spray it on the affected area, also you should start taking it by mouth. Start the standard protocol.

Can I use MMS on a radiation burn?

Q: Have you ever used MMS on a radiation burn? What do you suggest here?

A: I would use a drop of DMSO mixed with a drop of MMS that has been previously activated; put it on in a tiny spot, wait a few hours to see what happens in that spot, then the next time, cover a bigger area.

Does MMS need to be applied topically when treating keratosis or ingesting it will be enough? What is DMSO?

Q: What is the protocol for skin cancer – does it need to be applied topically or will ingesting it be enough? If so, what is the right dosage? What about precancerous spots called "keratosis"? Should they be treated topically? When you spoke of applying MMS topically to yourself and using DMSO – what is DMSO? And where can I find it?

A: DMSO is a material similar to kerosene in that it has a characteristic that allows it to soak into and through all body parts, and with it, it soaks the body cells and dissolves almost anything that's not a part of the cell, and then washes it out of the cell. It's been in use for the last 50 years in the US, and there are no bad results by DMSO, although the FDA said it cannot be used on humans. You can also spray MMS Topically. I use 20 drops of MMS, 100 drops of citric acid, and a 3 minute wait in a 2 ounce spray bottle. Spray the area several times a day and allow it to dry.

Can both precancerous spots (keratosis) and the Herpes Virus be treated successfully with MMS?

Q: As far as skin cancer goes - would precancerous spots (keratosis) respond to MMS, and would it need to be applied topically to work or is ingesting it enough?

With herpes virus, I was wondering if MMS actually eliminates the virus from the body (versus just eliminating or controlling an active outbreak)? Do you know of any cases where a person got a herpes blood test after treating with MMS and the test was negative?

A: For skin cancer. Mix one drop of MMS with 5 drops of lemon or citric acid solution and wait 3 minutes. Now, take 3 drops of that solution and add to 3 drops of DMSO and mix it together. Put it on the cancer immediately. If you need more than 3 drops, use four or five or more and always use the same number of DMSO drops. If it is cancer, it will begin to burn right away and the burning should not last long. Maybe 3 to 5 minutes. Once the burning has stopped, cover the area with Vaseline, and cover that with a bandage of some kind. The cancer should come out within a day or two. Do not pull it out. It might come out with the bandage. Make sure you get enough drops on it to kill it the first try, so when it starts to burn you could add a drop or two of MMS. Most skin cancers, however, are cured simply by taking MMS by mouth, but not always. If it burns but does not go away, it might be some form of fungus.

Generally herpes is one of the hardest things to handle but it can be handled. Just keep increasing the doses to at least 15 drops 3 times a day for a week or two, then check and verify your progress. If not, keep it up. It will eventually get it. We have heard of people feeling much better with MMS, but we do not have the before or after blood tests to make sure they are completely cured.

Will it help if I rinse my face with a solution of MMS in hopes of preventing the continued appearance of those precancerous keratoses?

Q: I was wondering was the efficacy or rinsing my face with a solution in hopes of preventing the continued appearance of those precancerous keratoses, or the disappearance of those that are already there…. Has anyone tried a mild solution in a small volume nebulizer for chronic asthma? Or will the internal solution help?

A: Get a small spray 2 ounce bottle mix 20 drops of MMS with 100 drops of citric acid solution, or lemon juice, wait 3 minutes and fill the rest of the 2 ounce bottle with water, spray it on 2 or 3 times a day and keep taking MMS by mouth. If the spray stings, then reduce the strength by pouring out ½ of the bottle and adding water. It can help asthma and so will taking it by mouth. Most asthma sufferers get relief and over time seem to be cured. The spray is a different strength than taking it by mouth.

Can MMS Help Extreme Skin Itching?

Q: I had surgery to fix hernias and when I got out of hospital my hands started itching and breaking out with bad pimples and it has spread all over both hands and the insides of my forearms. I have tried everything and the doctors do not help. Will this help me?

A: Take a 2 ounce bottle put 20 drops and 100 drops of citric acid wait 3 minutes add the water and the mixture to the bottle and spray it on the affected area, also you should start taking it by mouth. Start the standard protocol.

Strokes

What form/concentrate of DMSO would be used (or how) with a stroke?

Q: What form/concentrate of DMSO would be used (or how) with a stroke?

A: Use 90% DMSO or 99.9% DMSO.

299

Will **MMS** assist with diabetes, arthritis, stroke victims and constipation?

Q: Will MMS assist with diabetes, arthritis, stroke victims and constipation?

A: Yes it will help all of those conditions.

What is DMSO and where can I purchase it?

Q: My mother has had a couple of mild strokes and I heard that DMSO will help her. What is DMSO and where can I purchase it?

A: You can buy DMSO from a natural health food store. You can go to any search web page and type in DMSO.

Surgery

Do you caution against taking it in the case of transplant surgery. Do you have any reservations about its use after joint replacement?

Q: Do you caution against taking it in the case of transplant surgery. Do you have any reservations about its use after joint replacement?

A: It is ok to take MMS after having a surgery; it is best since you will recover a lot faster.

I am having a colonoscopy. Do you recommend I stop the MMS treatment just prior to and during the surgery and

recovery time? If so, when I re-start will I need to start from the beginning again?

Q: I am having a colonoscopy. Do you recommend I stop the MMS treatment just prior to and during the surgery and recovery time? If so, when I re-start will I need to start from the beginning again?

A: I would recommend that you do not stop taking MMS that is what will keep your infections down and it will make sure your recovery is much faster than normal.

Teeth and Mouth

Does MMS react with metal fillings?

Q: Does MMS react with metal fillings?

A: MMS does not react with metals of the mouth including mercury. It is a weak oxidizer and thus cannot oxidize these metals. Thus adds no additional metal contamination.

Can MMS take the infection out of a tooth?

Q: Can MMS take the infection out of a tooth? Do I understand correctly that bacteria, parasites and viruses that the MMS kills just oxidize? They leave to residue behind for the body to get rid of?

A: Yes it will clear the infection; in fact I know a lot of people who brush with MMS, just prepare it like a normal drink, like if you were going to drink it and then you brush your teeth. I

301

have a lot of success stories with gums and teeth and you are correct it does leave residue behind for the body to get rid of, but in the case of brushing you teeth the residue is a very small amount which you will wash out when you rinse you mouth.

Do I need to brush with baking soda after using MMS?

Q: Someone said we need to brush with baking soda after using MMS? Will there be a conflict if a person is also taking cumadin, lipitor or other RX including like leavaquin or cipro antibiotics?

A: You do not have to use baking soda after brushing with MMS. You use MMS as a normal tooth paste and you can also use it as a mouth wash. If the person is taking some kind of drug or medicine, just wait from 2 to 3 hours apart. MMS does not conflict with Medicines.

Can MMS be used as a mouth wash for gum disease and what would be the correct protocol?

Q: Can MMS be used as a mouth wash for gum disease and what would be the correct protocol?

A: Yes you can use MMS as a tooth paste and mouth wash, Make up a 10 drop solution as if you were going to drink it in other words add 50 drops of citric acid to the 10 drops of MMS wait the 3 minutes and half glass of water to that and by soaking your tooth brush in the solution, brush your teeth and gums 3 or 4 times a day use a soft tooth brush and after a week and see how your gums are doing.

Have you had any MMS customers with teeth problems, like needing a root canal? Can MMS be used as a mouthwash?

Q: Have you had any MMS customers have problems with their teeth, like needing a root canal? Can MMS be used as a mouthwash?

A: Of course, use it as a mouth wash. Make up a 6 or 8 drop dose as if you were going to take it and then use that as a mouth wash. Be sure to use the citric acid activator and the 3 minute wait. Brush your teeth with this solution several times a day at first, and then reduce to once a day. No matter how health you think your teeth are this will make them healthier.

Will MMS hurt dental fillings?

Q: I am so excited to begin this protocol for myself and my 11 year old daughter. However, I did see there are some things that need to be taken into account with dental fillings/crowns... Our appointment to remove the old materials via Huggins protocol with bio friendly materials is not until Nov 14th. Should we wait until after wards? Where can I get info on this?

A: MMS does not hurt dental work. Just do not leave it in the mouth for hours. If determined a method that people who have developed a tremendous aversion to MMS can use. It is not for the average MMS taker. It is only for those who just cannot take MMS otherwise. You daughter would benefit from having her mouth in better shape by the time she gets to the dentist. One should brush their teeth for 30 seconds with

MMS. It will not hurt the crowns and fillings. Then rinse your mouth with fresh water after 30 seconds.

How many times should I brush my teeth with the MMS and how much should I use to rinse my mouth if I have a bad toothache?

Q: I have two bad toothaches. How many times should I brush my teeth with the MMS and how much should I use to rinse my mouth?

A: Use 10 drops of MMS and 50 drops of citric acid, you can brush your teeth as many times as you like, you can also wash your mouth like a normal wash mouth using the same drops to citric acid ration do that 2 times a day.

Will MMS help me with Hypothyroidism resulting from sever dental infections that have been in my teeth and jaw bones for many years?

Q: I have been diagnosed with Hypothyroidism resulting from sever dental infections that have been in my teeth and jaw bones for many years. I have had 8 teeth removed and the infections scrapped out. But I am told I should have all my teeth removed and have my entire jawbone scarped out to clear all of the infection. I have been told my thyroid is destroyed and my immune system weak. I am very swollen with edema as a result of my bodies attempt to deal with all the remaining infections. Will the MMS help this situation?

A: First thing you need to do is overcome the infections in your mouth I do not think you need to have your teeth pulled, make up a 10 drop MMS solution add 50 drops of citric acid wait the 3 minutes add half a glass of water to that and by pour the solution on your toothbrush, brush your teeth 3 or 4 times a day brush your gums, use a soft toothbrush. After a week and see how your gums are doing, chances are they will be well in a week. Then do the standard protocol. Finally go to the health food store and buy some iodine solution and take up to 30 drops a day start at 2 drop and work your way up make sure your body gets saturated with iodine do not worry about over doing the iodine just go slow, increase slowly you need all of your organs saturated with iodine, finally begin getting off all the medication slowly.

Can I use MMS as a mouthwash or as toothpaste?

Q: Can I use MMS as a mouthwash or as toothpaste?

A: Yes you can use MMS as a tooth paste and mouth wash, Make up a 10 drop solution as if you were going to drink it in other words add 50 drops of citric acid to the 10 drops of MMS wait the 3 minutes and half glass of water to that and by soaking your tooth brush in the solution, brush your teeth and gums 3 or 4 times a day use a soft tooth brush. Also use it as a mouth wash what is left of the solution you can use it as a mouth wash.

Is MMS safe to use when you have metal under your crowns?

Q: I have just ordered a bottle of MMS but am reluctant to use it as still have some metal under my crowns - I cannot find the answer in your book is it safe to use?

A: MMS does not have enough power to oxidize metal or react with metal, so it is safe to use.

Can MMS take the infection out of a tooth?

Q: Can MMS take the infection out of a tooth? Do I understand correctly that bacteria, parasites and viruses that the MMS kills just oxidize? They leave to residue behind for the body to get rid of?

A: Yes it will clear the infection, in fact I know a lot of people who brush their teeth with MMS, and they just prepare it like a normal drink, like if they were going to drink it and then they brush their teeth. I have a lot of success stories with gums and teeth and you are correct it does leave residue behind for the body to get rid of.

I noticed the MMS stained my teeth a light brown in a few places?

Q: I noticed the MMS stained my teeth a light brown in a few places. I have not been to the dentist yet. Have you ever heard of this? Do you have any suggestions?

A: I have never heard of anyone's teeth turning light brown. For your information, there have been people who have brushed their teeth with MMS and their teeth feel much healthy and actually started to whiten up. What you can do is: Mix 10 drops of MMS with 50 drops of citric acid or lemon juice. You can brush your teeth with a gentle tooth brush, just dip it into the cup and brush your teeth. Do this 2 or 3 times a day, if you have some solution left over, you can use it as a mouth wash.

Why is MMS making my gums worse?

Q: Can you tell me why MMS may be making my gums worse (gum recession; teeth loose)? I am taking 10 MMS drops twice a day one hour apart with 50 drops of citric acid in each dose in a small amount of water and following up each with a glass of water.

A: What you need to do is mix a 10 drop dose of MMS which means 10 drops of MMS and 50 drops of lemon or citric acid, wait 3 minutes and add 4 ounce of water (1/2 glass water) use that to lightly brush your teeth and gums with in a week your teeth should be solidly in place and the infection should be gone. Your health starts at your mouth so start there. Thousands of people have made there mouth healthy by this method it should work for you in less than a week.

What is the protocol for gingivitis?

Q: What is the protocol for gingivitis?

A: The protocol for teeth make up a 10 drop solution as if you were going to drink it in other words add 50 drops of citric acid to the 10 drops of MMS wait the 3 minutes and add half glass of water to that and by pouring the solution on your tooth brush, brush your teeth 3 or 4 times a day after a week see how your gums and teeth are doing, chances are they will be well in a week or two.

Is it harmful to brush your teeth with MMS even though I

have mercury fillings?

Q: Is it harmful to brush your teeth with MMS even though I have mercury fillings?

A: Yes it is ok to use just mix ten drops of MMS and 50 drops of citric acid and soak your toothbrush in the solution and brush your teeth.

How many times a day should someone rinse their mouth out with MMS?

Q: I have been working with two people and the MMS - one is pretty straightforward – I am having her swish the solution of 6 drops with the citric acid in her mouth (instead of brushing) because she has a cyst like thing outside her gum. It's not exactly an abscess - they said they need to do surgery to fix the problem because it needs oxygen to dissipate. How many times a day do you think she should do that? I told her twice - but it's so tempting when you have that glass of liquid to not keep swishing - to just throw it down the sink. Also I also wanted to know what chemicals and minerals MMS was made of.

A: Well, if I were her I would swish four or five times a day. Nothing wrong with throwing the drink down the sink. Just make up a new batch in 3 hours or so. MMS is a chemical that generates chlorine dioxide when activated with lemon or lime juice. Chlorine dioxide is not chlorine. It does not resemble chlorine no more than table salt. Table salt is more than 1/2 chlorine. Do you see, just because it has the word chlorine does not make it the same as chlorine.

Can MMS help get rid of gingivitis? Will it harm any enamel that are in the teeth?

Q: Trying to get my wife to try brushing her teeth with MMS she is concerned because you caution not to allow the solution to remain in the mouth for more than 30 seconds. She has some concern that it could harm the enamel on her teeth. She does have a gingivitis problem and I assured her the MMS would help cure the problem. From my observation, in spite of a sometimes sweet tooth, she has always taken very good care of her teeth.

A: MMS will not harm the enamel. She can leave the solution in her mouth for an hour if she wants. I was just concerned with people being upset over the taste and not using it.

Do I have to brush with baking soda after using MMS?

Q: Someone said we need to brush with baking soda after using MMS?

A: You do not have to use baking soda after brushing with MMS. In fact it is better that you do not use baking soda as baking soda tends to neutralize the good effects of MMS. You can use MMS as a normal tooth paste and you can use it as a mouth wash as well.

How much stabilized oxygen should I use to treat a jaw infection?

Q: I live in South Africa and want to try this for a severe infection in my jaw (the bone, not the gums). I am trying to avoid surgery as my body is not strong enough to handle surgery at present. I do have stabilized oxygen at home and perhaps I could try it. How much should I use? I see you recommend 120 drops. Is there any reason why you sometimes recommend water instead of the fruit juice? I would prefer to use water as I have allergies to many things including most fruits.

A: The stabilized Oxygen might work. For this purpose, I would use about 40 drops. Add about 40 drops of lemon or lime juice, wait three minutes, then add about 1/2 glass of water (about 200 ml). I know the infection is in the jaw, but dip your tooth brush into the solution and brush your teeth and brush your gums. Take at least 5 minutes. Then swallow the remainder of the solution. Do this 4 or 5 or 6 times a day until the infection is gone. If you have true stabilized oxygen it will smell of chlorine after you add the lemon juice. It should say sodium chlorite on the side. The lemon juice is what makes the difference. It activates the stabilized oxygen.

Is it OK to use MMS if I have gold crowns in my mouth?

Q: I have written a message to you very recently about rinsing my mouth after using MMS. Another question surfaced in my mind about what will the solution do to my gold crowns? Will it be OK to use while gold crowns are in the mouth?

A: Make up a 10 drop solution as if you were going to drink it. In other words, add 50 drops of citric acid to the 10 drops of MMS, wait the 3 minutes, and add half glass of water to that. Pour the solution on your tooth brush, and brush your teeth and gums. You may also use it as a mouth wash.

Gold does not react. Anyone with any kind of metal in their mouth should get it replaced with non-metal. My friend just got his right molar gold filling replaced, and on the way home from the dentist, he regained sight in his right eye. It is ok. to use MMS in the mouth with metal fillings or crowns, but be sure to rinse the mouth with clean water after brushing.

Metal, even gold, creates a voltage in your mouth. Buy or borrow a voltmeter and put one electrode on the gold and one electrode touching the inside of your cheek. You will notice a as much as ½ volt being generated in your mouth. There is supposed to be no voltage there at all. That's the reason my friend regained his sight, the voltage was gone.

Has anybody tried injectable MMS or any protocol for tooth/gum/jaw abscess?

Q: Anybody tried injectable MMS for tooth/gum/jaw abscess? Any protocols available ? If not any suggestions? Thank you kindly!

A: No one has needed to use IV for tooth and mouth diseases, just brush your teeth with MMS and the abscesses that are not inside the tooth will be gone within hours. Make up a 10 drop solution as if you were going to drink it. In other words, add 50 drops of citric acid to the 10 drops of MMS. Wait 3 minutes and add half a glass of water. Pour the solution on your tooth brush and then brush teeth and gums 3 or 4 times a day. Remember to use a soft tooth brush. In the case of abscess anywhere except inside a tooth, the pain should go away within an hour or two. After a week, see how your gums are doing. Chances are they will be well. You can also use this solution as a mouth wash.

Is it true that I can use the MMS as a mouth wash to treat gum disease and periodontitis?

Q: I have just purchased some MMS primarily because I read that it was helpful in reversing gum disease and periodontitis, however I cannot relocate the information on the web relating to this particular issue, cannot remember which site it was on. Are you able to help point me in the correct direction? I think it said something about using MMS as a mouth wash?

A: Yes you can use MMS as a tooth paste and mouth wash. Make up a 10 drop solution as if you were going to drink it; in other words, add 50 drops of citric acid to the 10 drops of MMS, wait the 3 minutes and add half a glass of water to that. Soak your tooth brush in the solution, brush your teeth and gums 3 or 4 times a day, remember to use a soft tooth brush and after a week, see how your gums are doing. Chances are they will be well in a week. Also with what is left of the solution, use it as a mouth wash.

What is the best way to treat a tooth-gum condition if the gums seem to be receding?

Q: I have one client out of the many that treat themselves with MMS by now, that uses the MMS-SOLUTION exactly according to your protocol, but in her case, it so far seems to worsen the tooth-gum-condition.

The gums do look very healthy, maybe better than before even, but they are dramatically receding ! Do you have any comments on that ?

A: "Do the gums sting or pain when the MMS is applied? If they do, stop using the MMS immediately. Go to the health food store and buy some Aztec Clay. It comes in a jar in the powdered form. Use this clay to brush the teeth. Use it liberally and brush three of four times a day for a week or so. Brush and then rinse the mouth thoroughly. If the mouth is indeed getting worse, it is not a regular mouth type disease, it's worse. But the clay will kill it quickly.

So you have to determine (although the clay will not hurt in any case) that the mouth is getting worse. Just a little receding gums may be healthy.

Maybe those gums have been swollen for most of her life with a gum disease, and now that the disease is clearing out, the gums are receding to where they are supposed to be. Feel them. Are they good and hard? If they are, do not worry. In any case, better get the clay and make sure. Because the worse diseases that could be out there would be fungus and modern science has no cure for. Only the Aztec clay can do that.

How often should I brush my teeth with MMS for the relief of toothache?

Q: I have two bad toothaches. How many times should I brush my teeth with the MMS and how much should I use to rinse my mouth?

A: Use 10 drops of MMS and 50 drops of citric acid, to brush your teeth with as many times as you like.

You can also use the same MMS drops to citric acid ratio, to rinse your mouth out, just like a normal mouth wash, twice a day.

Thyroid

Will my thyroid medication interact with the MMS?

Q: I take thyroid medicine. In the morning and also bioidentical hormones as prescribed. I take one in the morning and one in the afternoon, but I will now take that one after dinner or before so as not to interact with the MMS. I take taurine and magnesium just before bed, is that OK to take with the MMS? Or should I take an hour before? Does it carry out the mercury or what?

A: I am glad you are starting MMS. It is best to separate MMS from all medicines you can. Separate them by 2 or 3 hours. MMS does not interfere with other medications, but it is best to separate them. MMS does carry out the mercury and removes heavy metal.

Does chlorine dioxide deplete iodine levels or affect the thyroid gland?

Q: I have been taking MMS for three weeks and am feeling very much better, however I have a question. Will the chlorine dioxide deplete the iodine and affect my thyroid gland?

A: Chlorine dioxide does not deplete iodine levels or affect your thyroid gland so you have nothing to worry about.

Toxins

Will MMS help rid my body of the toxins and heavy metals that are in my system from taking psychiatric drugs?

Q: Will MMS help rid my body of the toxins and heavy metals that are in my system from taking psychiatric drugs?

A: Normally it helps with psychiatric drugs, sometimes a little bit, and sometimes a lot, and sometimes not at all. About heavy metals: We tested people for heavy metals, then gave them the MMS, for a couple of weeks, and then tested them again and they tested free of the heavy metals. However, the test that we used was the roots of hairs pulled from the head. This is supposed to be a good test, but others have said that it is not a good test. Not all of the problems from drugs can be attributed to heavy metals, but we have had good results from the use of MMS with drugs. Just start at 1 drop or 1/2 drop and work one's way up by increasing 1 drop each day.

What toxins are washed away from the body using your MMS solution?

Q: What toxins are washed away from the body using your MMS solution?

A: MMS kills pathogens and oxidizes heavy metals, the body then washes away the residue. There is some evidence that MMS oxidizes other toxins, but I do not know which ones. However, what most people believe is caused by toxins is almost always caused by pathogens, often colonies of pathogens that are not known, but when they are killed many problems disappear.

Weight Problems

Will MMS help in weight loss? Will MMS effect or help the metabolism of the cells?

Q: Will MMS help in weight loss? Will MMS effect or help the metabolism of the cells?

A: There is some weight loss and it helps, but one needs a weight loss program in conjunction with the MMS. Do not know about the metabolism of the cells, but would imagine it helps. It helps to get rid of the virus, parasites, bacteria, yeast, and mold.

Have people been assisted in their weight issues through the use of MMS?

Q: Would you kindly tell me what other types of health issues have been "healed" using MMS? Have people been assisted in their weight issues?

So many people are obese these days that something like that would be amazing if it helped balance the acidity levels of the obese.

Please, share what you know, if anything about the possibilities of working with this category of ill health.

A: Some people have gotten some relief from overweight, but not a great deal so far. Who knows what might happen as we develop better protocols. But as it says in book 2, never assume that it will not help any condition. MMS is a killer. It kills pathogen, oxidizes heavy metals and most other poisons leaving the good bacteria and healthy cells untouched. Everyone has a viral load, and a bacteria load as well as a load of mold and yeast. Even if these anaerobic microorganisms do not cause disease, they can settle in many places and cause just plain old bad health. Once the MMS is thoroughly saturated the body, all that is gone, leaving a clean body without heavy metals.

MMS Protocols

How To Make MMS

What you will need to make 12.6 ounces of MMS

1. You will need at least a 15 ounce bottle. It can be clear plastic if you do not intend to keep the liquid in the bottle for more than a couple of days. This is OK if you are waiting to transfer the liquid to dark bottles or containers. Just be sure that you do not leave the liquid MMS in the clear bottle. You could actually get away with leaving it in a clear bottle if you kept the clear bottle in a closed tight cabinet. Do not leave it in a refrigerator as refrigerators are opened to the light too often.

2. At least one quart of distilled water. **Not** use any other kind of water. It's okay to used purified water if it says, "For all distilled water purposes." Do not use spring water of mineral water unless it is an emergency and you cannot wait.

3. A plastic pitcher that has a good pouring spout.

4. A one quart pan or larger that can be heated. Do not use metal including stainless steel. Use glass or Corning Ware or a new Teflon coated pot that does not have any scratches through to the metal.

319

5. Some kind of fairly accurate gram scale and must be accurate to 1/10 gram. An electronic postal scale will do. Postal spring scales would be okay if you had some accurate weights to adjust the scale with just before you use it.
6. A black marking pen.
7. Some small bottles to put the MMS solution in after you make it. pharmacies have small brown bottles with droppers. It's okay to use these bottles so long as you never allow the MMS solution to get up into the rubber bulb. If you tip the bottle over, remove the dropper and wash it out with water making sure the bulb is washed thoroughly.
8. You will need at least 100 grams of sodium chlorite. **Buying** this chemical make sure it is chlorite that you are buying and not chloride. Chloride will not work. You will notice that the sodium chlorite comes in flakes, either white or slightly yellow.

When buying sodium chlorite do not tell them what you are using it for. Tell them it is for water purification tests. The first thing that they will tell you is that their chemicals are not for internal use. That is not something to worry about. That is what all the sources of sodium chlorite specify, even those that sell their chemicals for public water systems.

Remember, when you add distilled water you are diluting the chemical. Then when you use only 12 drops and you dilute that with ½ glass of water or juice, any impurities are also diluted. By the time you have done that much dilution, the impurities are always way below the maximum allowable impurities per day that you can afford to put in your body. The sales people are always worried about being sued, so they will always try to talk you out of buying the chemical, or even refuse to sell it to you if you tell them what you are going to use it for.

Checking the sodium chlorite powder to make sure it is real. I worry that someone might try to fool you into thinking some other powder is sodium chlorite in order to make you fail at curing someone, or just some clerk might be too dumb to sell you the correct powder. So here is how you check to make sure that you absolutely have the correct powder. First you must buy the strips that test for chlorine from any swimming pool store.

(1)When you open your package the sodium chlorite must be flaky. Several companies have sold sodium chlorite that is not flaky in the last couple of years. If there is no flakes assume that you do not have sodium chlorite, but go ahead and do the other steps given here. If the chemical passes the following tests it is indeed sodium chlorite and they, for some reason, ground the flakes before you got it.

(2)Crush up a few of the flakes into powder. (Do this by putting the flakes into a tablespoon and crushing with a second spoon).

(3)Put ½ teaspoon of the crushed powder into an empty glass and add three level teaspoons of distilled water. Swirl gently until the powder is completely dissolved in the water. You could warm slightly to aid in dissolving or you could heat the three teaspoons of water before adding to the powder.

(4)Now drop 10 drops of this solution into an empty glass.

Add ½ teaspoon of vinegar. Any vinegar will do as long as it says "5% acetic acid" or "5% acidity." Wait three minutes.

(5)Wet a pool chlorine strip with this solution. It should read at least 1 ppm chlorine present. It is actually reading chlorine dioxide (pool chlorine strips cannot tell the difference).

(6)Now wet a second pool chlorine indicator strip with the original solution from which you took the 10 drops. This solution should read no more or less than the above (5) test. If your powder fails either step 5 or step 6 you do not have sodium chlorite powder. Someone is fooling you or they have made a mistake. Run the test one more time to make sure. If it does not pass the test, do not use it. If your powder is okay, follow the steps given.

Making the MMS solution: MMS solution is 28% sodium chlorite powder. The 100 grams is 28% of 357 grams. That is 12.6 ounces. If you buy a bottle of 100 grams, you should just check that it indeed has 100 grams in it before adding it to the solution.

Step 1: Verify that 100 grams or 3.54 ounces is contained in your bottle of sodium chlorite.

Step 2: out nine ounces of distilled water and add it to your heating pot. Be very careful to get nine ounces exactly.

Step 3: dump the 3.54 ounces (the 100 grams) of sodium chlorite into the 9 ounces of water in the heating pot. The heating pot should not be on the fire yet. Put the heating pot on the hot plate and stir until dissolved. Once the white flakes or powder is dissolved immediately remove it from the fire. It should never be heated to the boiling point. It should only be warm when the sodium chlorite is finally dissolved.

Never go away and leave it heating. It dissolves fast. Stay and stir until dissolved.

Step 4: liquid should be yellow and clear. Pour into the pitcher and then use the pitcher to pour into your plastic container with a lid. Put the lid on and set aside to cool. **Warning:** when the MMS is spilled on a table or on the floor it must be cleaned up with plenty of water. Never allow it to dry. The white powder is very flammable when dry.

Step 5: dark colored bottles, preferably glass bottles and transfer from your original bottle. Label and date your bottles. The MMS lasts for several years. It should have maximum data on the label for someone a couple of years from now who might want to use it. For example, if a hurricane damaged much of your home and help was days away, if the bottle had proper information it could be used to help you or save your life. If it was just a dark bottle with no label, no one would know to use it.

Quick tip: 100 ml of MMS Should weigh 122grams. So go get a good gram scale and check your formula for accuracy.

Make 50% Citric Acid Solution

You will need a good food grade citric acid and distilled or purified water.

Always measure equal amounts of water and citric acid, combine in a clean bowl or container and stir until dissolved. Refrigerate your solution for a longer shelf life.

Make a pH Booster

1. Start with one liter (33.8 ounces) of distilled or purified water.
2. Add 3 drops of MMS (unactivated, only use the MMS with NO activator)
3. Stir with plastic spoon and your water is ready to use.

Where To Get Supplies

Sodium Chlorite Flakes

Most places will require some type of business license to acquire this product. As of the printing of this book you can get this item at the following places online without a license: http://www.sodiumchlorite.ca/

Do a search... There may be more suppliers.

Citric Acid

Your local health food store usually carries this. You can also buy this item online, just do a search.

Distilled Water

Walmart and grocery stores carry distilled water in the water section.

Ready to use MMS Solution and Activator

USA Suppliers

Dennis Richard MMS Dr.
http://www.mmsdr.com
760-536-6123

Keavy's Corner
http://keavyscorner.com
E-Mail: Sales@Keavyscorner.com
Toll Free - (1 888 751 4964) Retail and Wholesale MMS and
Sodium Chlorite. Bulk Sales available. Calcium
Hypochlorite, DMSO, Living Clay

Mineral-Solutions.Net
http://www.Mineral-Solutions.net
E-Mail: Sales@Mineral-Solutions.Net

MMS1 and MMS2
Subtle Energy Therapy
http://www.SubtleEnergyTherapy.org
800-581-1948

Project Greenlife International
http://www.ProjectGreenLife.com
888-349-9428

MMS Wholesale
jimbenner@sbcglobal.net
888-839-6007

Mountain Well-Being
http://www.mountainwellbeing.com
828-658-4237

Merril Anderson
937-879-0402

Miracle Mineral
http://buymiraclemineral.com
800-921-4528

The Incredible Earth
http://www.TheIncredibleEarth.com
877-427-7704 Toll Free

MMS Suppliers in Argentina

Luis Garcia
http://www.MMS-AR.com.ar
E-Mail: info@mms-ar.com.ar

MMS Suppliers in Australia

Alison Cousland
http://www.MiracleMineralSolutions.com
Skype: "AllyInSpirit"

Miracle MS
http://www.MiracleMS.com
03-9737-0807

MMS Protocols

Miracle Supplement
http://www.MiracleSupplement.com.au

The MMS Experience
http://www.TheMMSExperience.com.au
0409995738

MMS Australia Wholesale / Retail
http://www.mmsaustralia.co.za
0409995738

Kim Wheaton
gone.cruising@bidpond.com
0409995738

Miracle Mineral Supplement Russel Perry
Http://www.MiracleMineralSupplement.com.au
0419-179-389

MMS Suppliers in Austria

LuxusLine LTD.
http://www.Mineral-MMS.eu

MMS Suppliers in Brazil

MMS Brazil
http://www.MiracleMineral.com.br
55-35-9819-0072

MMS Suppliers in British Isles

Subtle Energy Therapy
http://www.SubtleEnergyTherapy.com.uk

MMS Suppliers in Canada

MMS Supplier in British Columbia
http://www.MMSSupplier.com
Victoria B.C.

MMS Supplier in Ontario
http://www.MMSMiracle.com/Canada
mms_canada@rogers.com

Canada's Subtle Energy Therapy MMS1 & MMS2
http://www.Health4AllInfo.ca
780-634-8950 - Rev. Denis Korski, D.MMS

Home Products Store
http://www.MiracleMineralSupplement.ca
403-652-1655

Deana Whitely
dd22@lincsat.com

MMS Suppliers in Colombia

MMS Colombia
http://www.mmscolombia.com
info@mmscolombia.com

MMS Protocols

MMS Suppliers in Czech Republic, Slovakia

Suppliers in Slovakia Z Technology
http://www.eMMS.cz
E-Mail: info@eMMS.cz
775-734-829
776-601-571

MMS Suppliers in Denmark

Alma-Senteret As
http://www.AlmaSenteret.com

MMS Suppliers in Dominican Republic

MMS For Hispaniola
http://www.MMSforHispaniola.com
E-Mail: musicachica@hotmail.com
829-491-3688

MMS Suppliers in England

Mineral Solutions NET
http://www.Mineral-Solutions.net
E-Mail: Sales@Mineral-Solutions.Net

MMS Suppliers in France

Tout le MMS en Francais
http://www.MMSFrance.com
Telechargement des livres MMS en Francais Vente de Produits

MMS en Francais
Editions Mediacore France Livres, DVDs, Videos, News Jim
Humble,Adam Abrahams

http://www.MMSJimHumble.fr

http://www.Comprende-Le-MMS.fr

Monde & Afrique Francophone: E-mail(voir site)ou Tele:00 33
(0)5 49 86 58 00

MMS Suppliers in Germany

Arcadia Eden
http://www.Arcadia-Eden.de
0044-208-123-9492
0049-8856-80-30-848

Vitalundfitmit100
http://www.Vitalundfitmit100.de
00492166998066

MMS Suppliers in Haiti

MMS For Hispaniola
http://www.MMSforHispaniola.com
E-Mail: musicachica@hotmail.com
829-491-3688

MMS Suppliers in Hungary

Zapper Technology
http://www.e-MMS.hu

MMS Protocols

E-Mail: MMSHungary@gmail.com
+36-30-524-6850

MMS Suppliers in Iceland

Alma-Senteret As
http://www.AlmaSenteret.com

MMS Suppliers in Italy

Gianni
http://www.MiracleMineral.it
E-Mail: info@MiracleMineral.it
015-748346

MMS Suppliers in Mexico

MMS Mexico
http://www.MMSMexico.com.mx
52-662-301-09-93

MMS Suppliers in Nambia

H. Martine
E-Mail: Hildegard.Martine@gmail.com
+264-61-213014

MMS Suppliers in Netherlands

Roel Nulpont Groep
E-Mail: rs@nulpuntenergie.net

Nulpont Groep Health Practitioner Biophoton Therapy
E-Mail: ron@nulpuntenergie.net
Working with MMS since 2007. By energizing the MMS with
biophotons it becomes more potent.

MMS Suppliers in New Zealand

Even Keel Limited
http://www.EvenKeel.co.nz
07-858-4509

MMS New Zealand
http://www.MMSNewZealand.co.nz
E-Mail: info@MMSNewZealand.co.nz

Miracle Mineral
http://www.MiracleMineral.co.nz
info@miraclemineral.co.nz

MMS Suppliers in Norway

Alma-Senteret As
http://www.AlmaSenteret.com

MMS Suppliers in Poland

Wydawnictwo David
http://www.MiracleMineralPolska.pl
We offer MMS-book in Polish and ship worldwide.

MMS Suppliers in Portugal

MMS Protocols

Vital y en Forma con 100
http://www.Miracle-Mineral-Supplement.eu

MMS Suppliers in Spain

Vital y en Forma con 100
http://www.Miracle-Mineral-Supplement.es
003-497-134-3623

LuxusLine LTD,.
http://www.Mineral-MMS.com

MMS Suppliers in Sweden

Alma-Senteret As
http://www.AlmaSenteret.com

MMS Suppliers in MMS Suppliers in Africa / Southern African Regions / Indian Ocean Islands

Sommex (Pty) Ltd MMS - Wholesale/Retail Whole of Africa, Middle East + Indian Ocean Islands
E-Mail: sommex@iafrica.com
+27-11-791-1947
+27-0-834-538-566

MMS Suppliers in Thailand

Mineral-Solutions.Net
http://www.Mineral-Solutions.Net

Thomas Husted
E-Mail: ThomasHusted@Yahoo.com
"Our MMS comes in a high quality glass dropper bottle"

MMS Protocols

Alphabetical Index

MMS Protocols

Notes

Book Two

Notes

MMS Protocols

Notes

Notes

MMS Protocols

Notes